Basic Urological Management

Sanchia S. Goonewardene • Peter Pietrzak
David Albala

Basic Urological Management

Springer

Sanchia S. Goonewardene
East of England Deanery
Southend University Hospital
London
UK

Peter Pietrzak
Southend University Hospital NHS
Foundation Trust
Southend
UK

David Albala
Associated Medical Professionals
Syracuse
NY
USA

ISBN 978-3-319-98719-4 ISBN 978-3-319-98720-0 (eBook)
https://doi.org/10.1007/978-3-319-98720-0

Library of Congress Control Number: 2018959561

This Springer imprint is published by the registered company Springer Nature Switzerland AG
The registered company address is: Gewerbestrasse 11, 6330 Cham, Switzerland

Preface

Welcome to *Basic Urological Management*. We hope you enjoy and learn from this book. The aim of this book is to not only gain knowledge but an understanding of patient pathways and what to do next for patients at different steps in each pathway. It is perfectly fine not to know something in medicine and then to go and study about a topic or area. It is how we evolve our knowledge. The key is to study it in detail and then apply that knowledge to each clinical situation.

Everyone, at some point, has been at the start of their career. As a young doctor, I often had a difficult time, with consultants who expected a CCT level of knowledge, prior to gaining a training number. A few situations in particular stood out in my mind, where a knowledge of patient pathways or what to do in each specific clinic scenario would have helped. I had been through the library of textbooks to no avail. I needed a practical book that told me what to do and when.

It was in that job that I started to write. The first thing I wrote was a list of clinical management scenarios; it would be good to be aware of those scenarios as a junior doctor. This book is written entirely from that. In the words of one of my favourite consultants, 'You have to learn to cut your teeth somewhere.' (You have to start somewhere.) Work and train hard, and treat your patients as if they were family, and you will succeed.

London, UK — Sanchia S. Goonewardene
Southend, UK — Peter Pietrzak
Syracuse, NY, USA — David Albala

Acknowledgements

For my family and friends, for always supporting me in what I do.

For my team at Springer, for always giving me a chance to get published.

For Gladstone's Library, for always giving me a sanctuary in which to write.

For my mentor, anchorman and editor-in-chief, David Albala (credit for illustrations goes to him).

For my amazing crew at Southend, Peter Pietrzak, Pete Acher and Sampi Mehta.

For East of England Deanery and my TPD, Mr Oliver Wiseman (Winner of the Silver Cystoscope for Best Trainer), for always supporting me and my academic endeavours.

Contents

Abbreviations

AAA	Abdominal aortic aneurysm
AAST	American Association for the Surgery of Trauma
ADH	Antidiuretic hormone
A+E	Accident and emergency
AMH	Asymptomatic microhematuria
ATLS	Advanced Trauma Life Support
AUA	American Urological Association
AVM	Arteriovenous malformation
BCG	Bacillus Calmette-Guerin
BD	Twice daily
BP	Blood pressure
BPH	Benign prostatic hypertrophy
BXO	Balanitis xerotica obliterans
CCF	Congestive cardiac failure
CIS	Carcinoma in situ
CT	KUB Computed tomography of kidneys, ureters and bladder
CT IVU	Computed tomography intravenous urogram
CKD	Chronic kidney disease
Cr	Creatinine
CXR	Chest radiograph
CXM	Crossmatch
DRE	Digital rectal examination
DM	Diabetes mellitus
DI	Diabetes insipidus
EAU	European Association of Urology
ED	Erectile dysfunction
EGFR	Estimated glomerular filtration rate
ESWL	Extracorporeal shockwave lithotripsy
FFP	Fresh frozen plasma
FBC	Full blood count
Fr	French
FSH	Follicle-stimulating hormone
GA	General anaesthesia
G+S	Group and save

GU	Genitourinary
HB	Haemoglobin
HD	Haemodynamically
HOLEP	Holmium Laser Enucleation of the Prostate
HPCR	High-pressure chronic retention
HPV	Human papillomavirus
ICIQ-SF	International Consultation on Incontinence Questionnaire – Short Form
IIEF	International Index of Erectile Function
ISC	Intermittent self-catheterisation
IVC	Inferior vena cava
IVI	Intravenous infusion
IV	Intravenous
IVU	Intravenous urogram
IPSS	International Prostate Symptom Score
LA	Local anaesthesia
LFTs	Liver function tests
LH	Luteinising hormone
LHRH	Luteinising hormone-releasing hormone
LPCR	Low-pressure chronic retention
LTC	Long-term catheter
LUTS	Lower urinary tract symptoms
MAG 3	Nuclear Medicine MAG 3 Renogram
MC+S	Microscopy, culture and sensitivity
MDT	Multidisciplinary team meeting
MAG	Mercaptoacetyltriglycine
MIBC	Muscle-invasive bladder cancer
MRI	Magnetic resonance imaging
MS	Multiple sclerosis
NBM	Nil by Mouth
NICE	National Institute for Clinical Excellence
NMIBC	Non-muscle-invasive bladder cancer
Na	Sodium
NSAIDs	Nonsteroidal anti-inflammatory drug
NVH	Non-visible haematuria
OAB	Overactive bladder
Obs	Observations
OD	Once daily
OPA	Outpatient appointment
OPD	Outpatient department
PIRADS	Prostate Image Reporting and Data System
PPI	Proton-pump inhibitor
PSA	Prostate-specific antigen
PCNL	Percutaneous nephrolithotomy
PUJO	Pelviureteric junction obstruction

PV	Per vaginum
PVR	Post-void residual
Pt	Patient
Qmax	Maximum flow rate
RCC	Renal cell carcinoma
RESP	Rate Respiratory rate
Sats	Saturation
SCC	Squamous cell carcinoma
SHBG	Sex hormone-binding globulin
SHIM	Sexual Health Inventory for Men
SIRS	Systemic inflammatory response syndrome
SIADH	Syndrome of inappropriate antidiuretic hormone secretion
SPC	Suprapubic
STIs	Sexually transmitted infection
T stage	Tumour staging for cancer
TIS	Tumour in situ
TED	Thromboembolic device
TB	Tuberculosis
TCC	Transitional cell carcinoma
TFTs	Thyroid function tests
TURBT	Transurethral resection of the bladder tumour
TURP	Transurethral resection of the prostate
TOT	Transobturator tape
TVT	Transvaginal tape
TWOC	Trial without catheter
U+Es	Urea and electrolytes
USS	Ultrasound scan
USS KUB	Ultrasound scan of kidneys, ureters and bladder
UTI	Urinary tract infection
UV	Ultraviolet
VUR	Vesicoureteric reflux
WCC	White cell count

1 Visible Haematuria

Referral criteria

- As per NICE Guideance NG12, 2011.
- Aged 45 or over: unexplained visible haematuria without UTI.
- Visible haematuria that persists or recurrs after UTI treatment.
- Non visible haematuria and either dysuria or raised WCC.
- See patient as Target in haematuria clinic - 2 week wait (NICE Guidance).

Causes

- As per AUA guidelines, look for a cause:
- Neoplastic (renal cancer, urothelial cancer, bladder cancer (TCC-most common, SCC or adenocarcinoma), prostate cancer).
- Infection: UTI, cystitis, prostatitis.
- Inflammation-insertitial cystitis.
- Stones (renal, ureteric, bladder).
- Trauma (renal, ureteric, bladder, prostate or urethra).
- Nephrological: Intrinsic renal disease, nephropathies.
- Blood dyscracias and anticoagulation.
- Benign Prostatic Hyperplasia - large vascular prostate.
- Visible haematuria can indicate bleeding or clots from anywhere in the urinary tract.

S. S. Goonewardene et al., *Basic Urological Management*,
https://doi.org/10.1007/978-3-319-98720-0_1

History

- A comprehensive patient history is mandatory, EAU Guidelines, 2018.
- History: Extent and duration of haematuria, position in stream.
- UTIs, STIs, LUTS.
- Abdominal pain - look for stones/ infection/ clot colic/ tumour.
- Red flags: weight loss, bony aches, backache.
- Travel history: any recent foreign travel abroad - schistosoma/ TB.
- Past urological history: stones, trauma, cancer. Prior urological/ haematuria investigations. Even if investigated previously for haematuria, repeat investigations.
- Anticoagulation therapy.
- Prior bladder/ prostate radiotherapy.
- Risk factors: smoking, dyes, aromatic amines, hydrocarbons, occupation (Hairdressers).

Examination

- As per NICE Guidance on cancer recognition and referral.
- General exam- pallor, haemodynamic stability.
- Abdomen: palpable masses in flanks (renal mass), flank tenderness (stones). SPC mass (bladder mass or retention).
- Review of extermal genitatia with a chaperone (testicular tumour, epididymoorchitis or penile cancer), review of glans (CIS, penile SCC).
- PV- make sure the patient is consented for this (to see if the bladder is fixed, cervical tumours).
- DRE: size, consistency, firmness of prostate gland (prostate cancer), nodular prostate (BPH) ? boggy prostate (prostatitis, abcess).

Investigations

- As per EAU Guidelines on Investigation of bladder cancer:
- Urine dip and culture- if urine dip positive, patient cannot have flexible cystosocpy- send off MC+S and treat infection with region specific antibiotics.
- Bloods including renal function pre scan- EGFR >30 required. Also FBC (HB).
- Urine cytology- detects 90% of high risk cases and 10 % of low risk cases. This in contraversial, but most useful for established bladder cancer follow-up.
- CT IVU if EGFR >30 (to review upper tracts and look for filling defects).
- Flexible cystoscopy: conducted under LA, via aseptic technique. Zero degree lense to view inside of bladder- aim- identfy bladder tumour, usually TCC.

Outcome

- Identify patient performance status, fitness for anaesthetic and surgery.
- If bladder tumour is identified- for TURBT as target patient - histology is needed as first line management.
- Make sure the patient has a CT IVU if EGFR >30, and a CT chest for completion if muscle invasive.
- If there is a red patch on cystoscopy, for GA rigid cystoscopy and biopsy.
- If RCC or upper tract TCC identified or cytology positive, for renal MDT regarding ureteroscopy, nephrectomy or nephrouretrectomy.
- If stones identified- stone MDT for surveillance, ESWL, PCNL, or Ureteroscopy as appropriate.

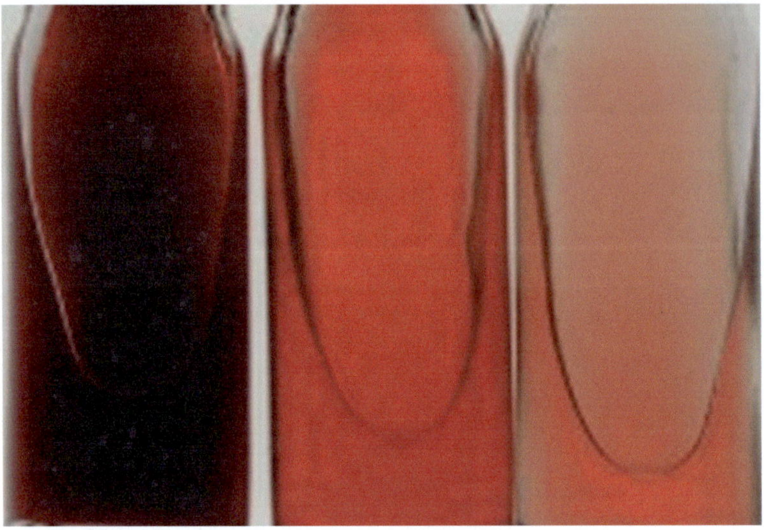

Fig. 1.1 Haematuria- from dark haematuria to light rose

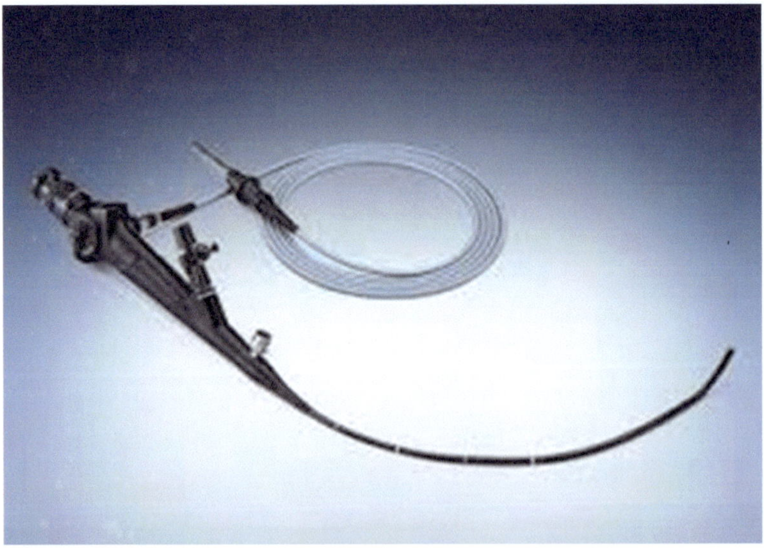

Fig. 1.2 Flexible cystoscopy kit- you will need a light source, giving set and saline to go with the scope. Part of haematuria assessment

Suggested Reading

AUA Guidelines on Diagnosis, Evaluation and Follow-up of Asymptomatic Microhematuria (AMH) in Adults, 2016.

EAU Guidelines on None Muscle Invasive Bladder Cancer, 2018.

NICE Guidance on Cancer Recgonition and Referral, NG12, 2011.

2 Diagnostic Pathway for Haematuria

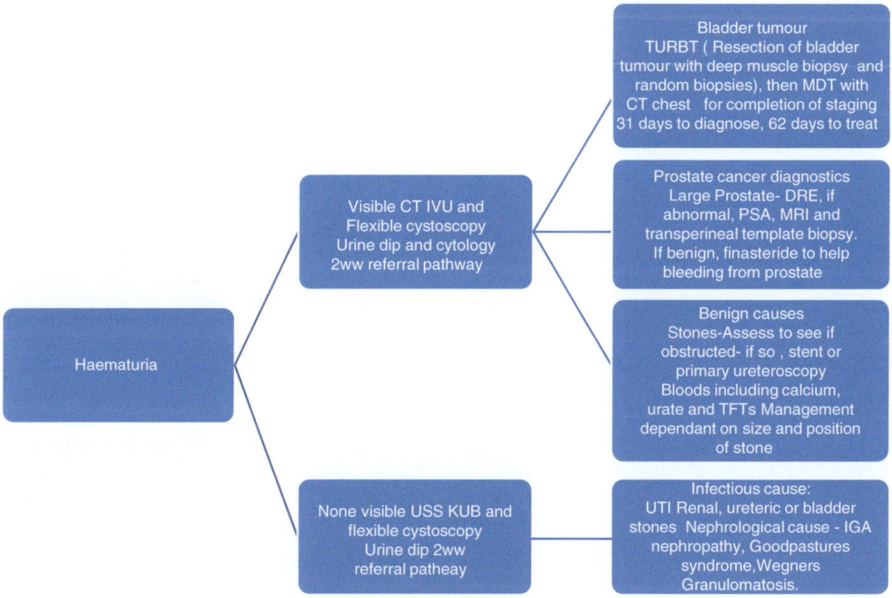

S. S. Goonewardene et al., *Basic Urological Management*,
https://doi.org/10.1007/978-3-319-98720-0_2

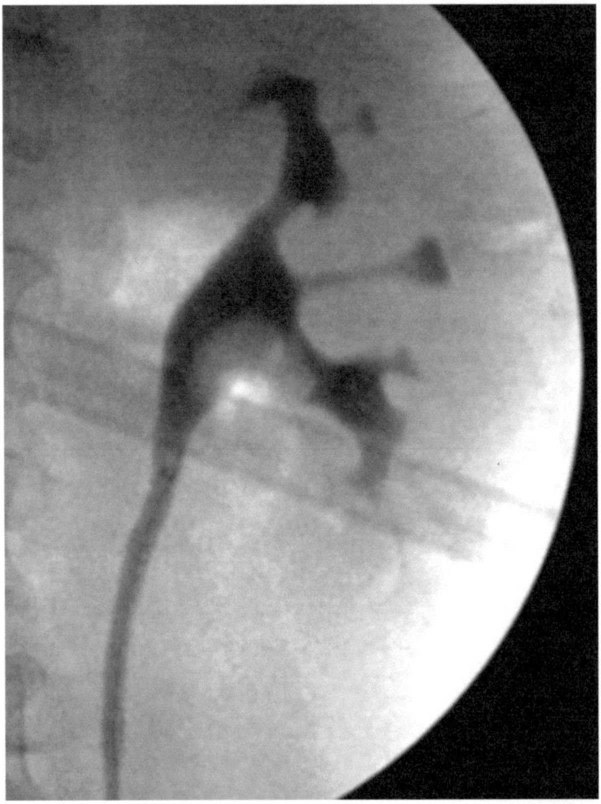

Fig. 2.1 An upper tract TCC on IVU

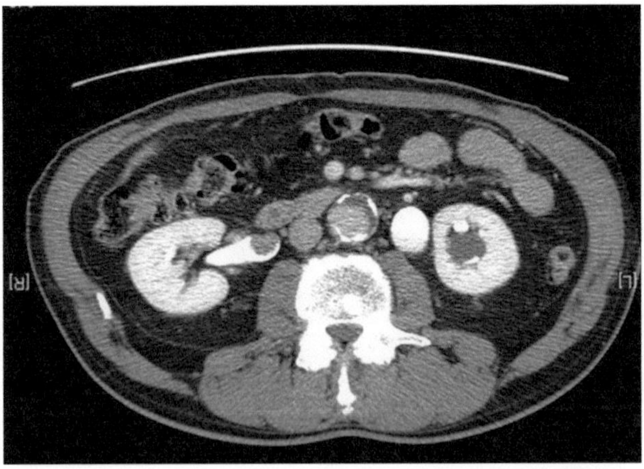

Fig. 2.2 An upper tract TCC on CT Urogram

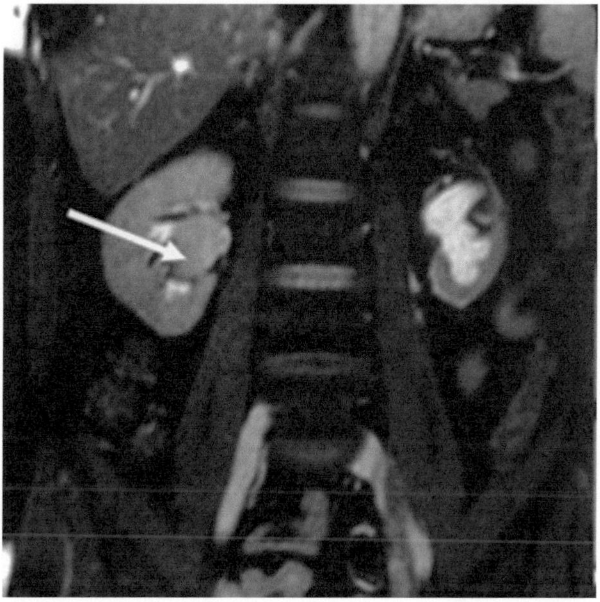

Fig. 2.3 An MRI demonstrating upper tract TCC

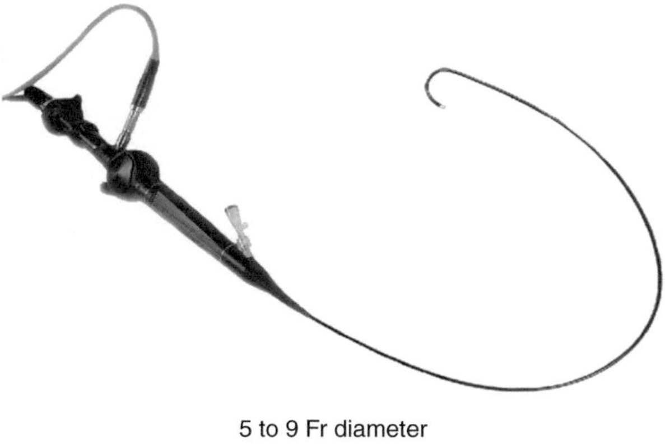

Fig. 2.4 A ureteroscope, to investigate upper tract TCC

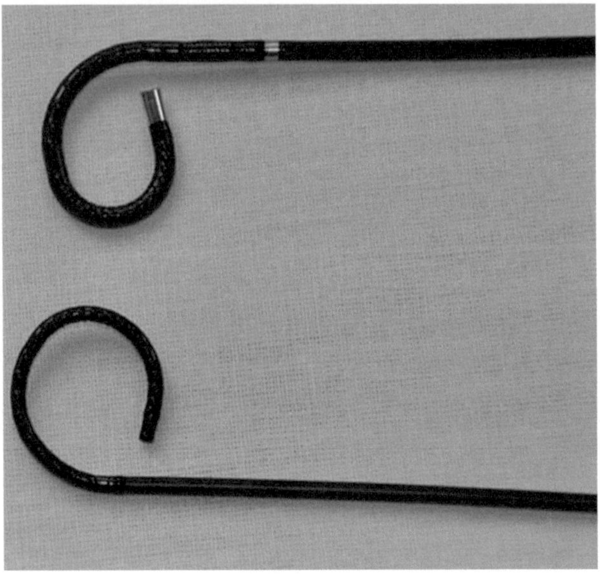

Fig. 2.5 Demonstrating tip deflection of ureteroscopes

Suggested Reading

AUA Guidelines on Diagnosis, Evaluation and Follow-up of Asymptomatic Microhematuria (AMH) in Adults, 2016.

EAU Guidelines on None Muscle Invasive Bladder Cancer and Muscle Invasive Bladder Cancer, 2018.

NICE Guidance on Cancer Recognition and Referral, NG12, 2011.

3 Non-Visible Haematuria

Referral criteria

- See patient as Target in haematuria clinic.
- 2 week wait, NICE Guidance, 2011.
- Haematuria (non-visible and unexplained) with dysuria or raised white cell count on a blood test, 60 and over.
- None urgent referral-people aged 60 and over with recurrent or persistent unexplained urinary tract infection.
- 90% of cases will have no underlying pathology.

Causes

- AUA Guidelines, 2016 specify to look for a cause.
- Causes:
- Infection: UTI, cystitis, prostatitis.
- Inflammation- insertitial cystitis.
- Stones (renal, ureteric, bladder).
- Trauma (renal, ureteric, bladder, prostate or urethra).
- Cancer (renal cancer, urothelial cancer, bladder cancer (TCC or SCC), prostate cancer).
- Intrinsic renal disease, nephropathies, CKD, nephrological causes, hypertension.
- Blood dyscrias and anticoagulation.
- BPH-large vascular prostate.

S. S. Goonewardene et al., *Basic Urological Management*,
https://doi.org/10.1007/978-3-319-98720-0_3

History

- A focused history is key. EAU Guidelines, 2018.
- History: Extent and duration of haematuria, other causes (UTIs, STIs, LUTS/ Retention)
  Red flags: weight loss bony aches backache, chest symptoms.
- Travel history: any recent foreign travel abroad- schistosoma/ TB.
- Past urological history: stones, trauma, cancer.
- Risk factors: smoking, dyes, aromatic amines, hydrocarbons.

Examination

- Abdomen: pallor, haemodynamic stability, palpable masses in flanks (renal mass), flank tenderness (stones), SPC mass (bladder mass or retention).
- Review of extermal genitatia with a chaperone (testicular tumour, epididymo-orchitis or penile cancer), review of glans (CIS, penile SCC).
- Per Vaginal Examination - make sure the patient is consented for this and you are chaperoned (to see if the bladder is fixed, cervical tumours, gynaecological malignancies).
- DRE: size, consistency, firmness of prostate gland (prostate cancer), nodular prostate (BPH), tender/ boggy prostate (prostatitis, abcess).

Investigations

- As per EAU Guidlines, 2018.
- Urine dip and culture- if urine dip positive, patient cannot have flexible cystosocpy- send off MC+S and treat infection with region specific antibiotics.
- Renal function and FBC (HB).
- Urine cytology.
- USS KUB: USS examination of kidneys, ureter and bladder.
- Flexible cystoscopy: conducted under LA, via aseptic technique. Zero degree lense to view inside of bladder- aim- identfy bladder TCC.

Suggested Reading

AUA Guidelines on Diagnosis, Evaluation and Follow-up of Asymptomatic Microhematuria (AMH) in Adults, 2016.
EAU Guidelines on None Muscle Invasive Bladder Cancer, 2018.
NICE Guidance on Cancer Recognition and Referral, NG12, 2011.

4 Management Pathway for Bladder Tumour

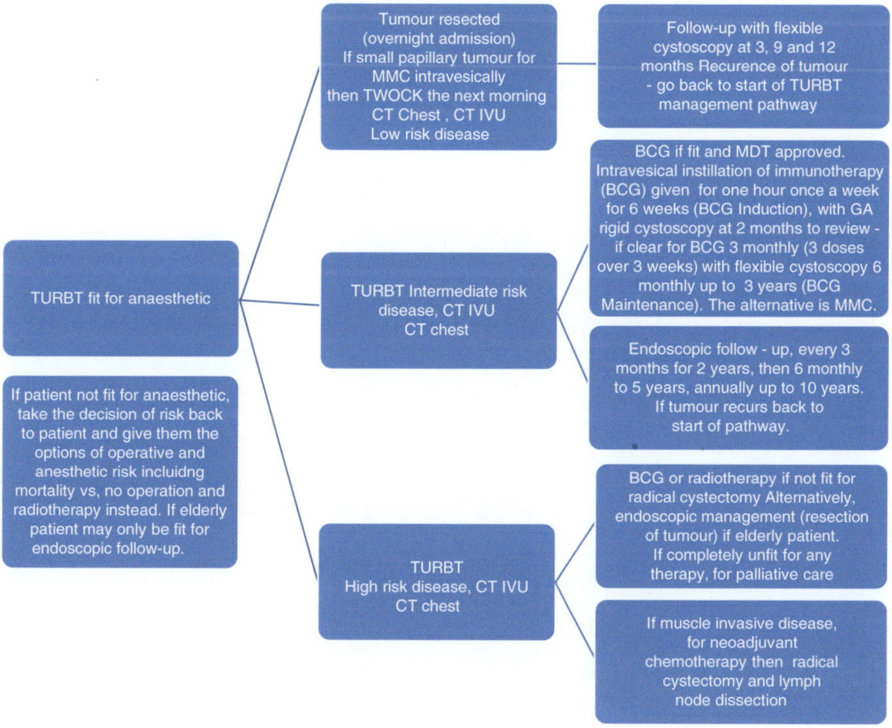

S. S. Goonewardene et al., *Basic Urological Management*,
https://doi.org/10.1007/978-3-319-98720-0_4

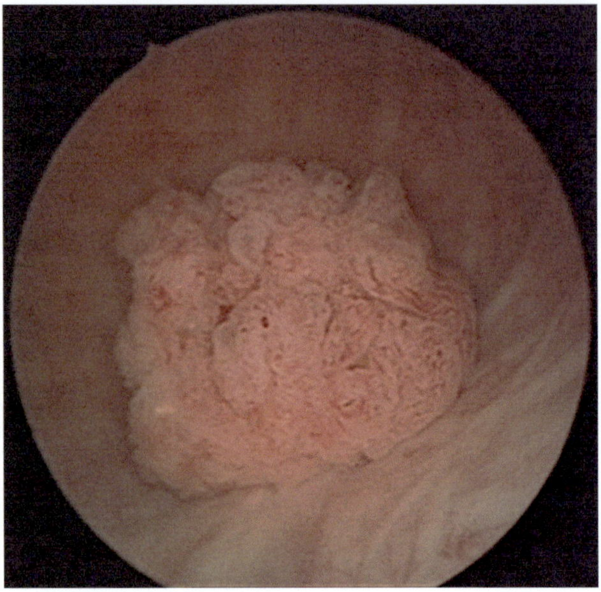

Fig. 4.1 Bladder tumour—a papillary and solid TCC

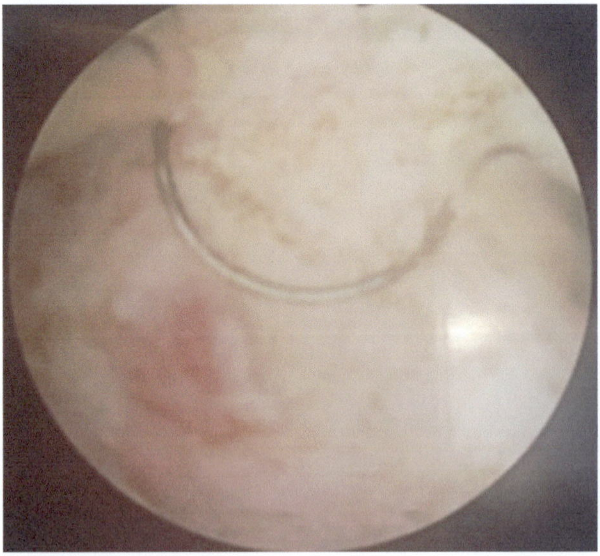

Fig. 4.2 Identifying ureteric orifice during tumour resection

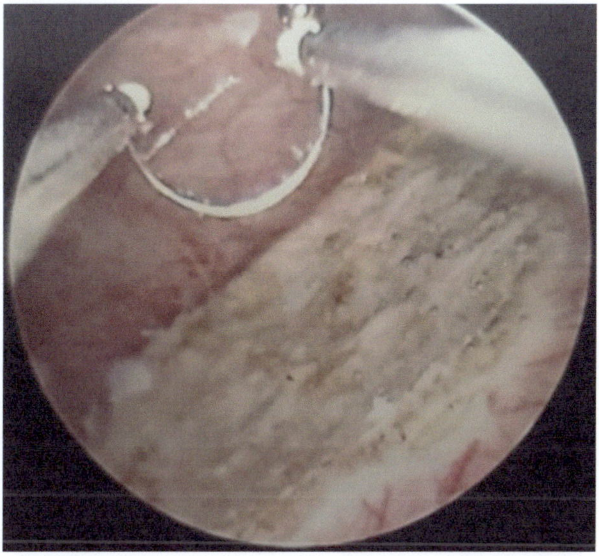

Fig. 4.3 Bladder base after tumour resection

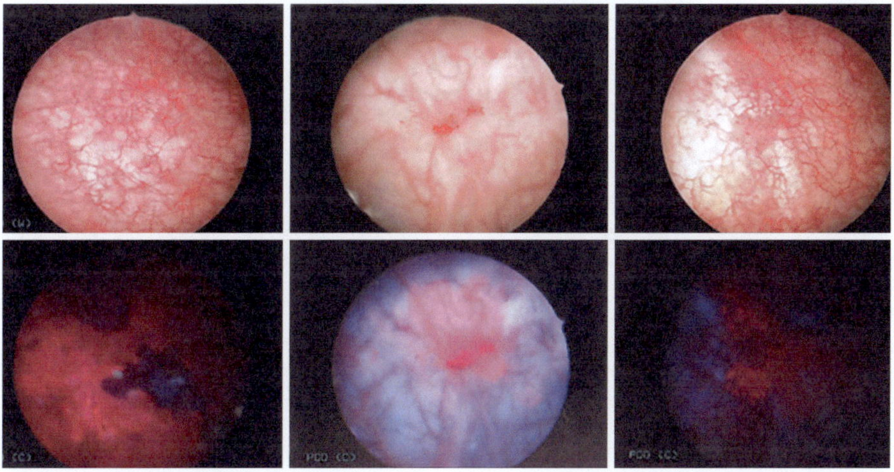

Fig. 4.4 Demonstrating blue light- hexyl- aminolevulinate gives off fluorescence under blue light allowing detection of bladder tumours

Suggested Reading

AUA Guidelines on Asymptomatic Microscopic Haematuria, 2016.
EAU Guidelines on None Muscle Invasive Bladder Cancer, 2018.
EAU Guidelines on Muscle Invasive Bladder Cancer, 2018.
NICE Guidelines Bladder Cancer Diagnosis and Management, 2015.

5 Elevated PSA/Abnormal DRE

Referral criteria

- PSA elevated according to age specific criteria.
- PSA is a 32 KD serine protease that liquifies the seminal ejaculate.
- The exact purpose is unknown.
- If the DRE is abnormal, or PSA elevated, refer patient to hospital as a 2 week wait patient. NICE Guideline, NG2.
- There is no evidence for PSA screening below the age of 54 routinely. AUA guidelines, 2013.
- If a patient has a strong family history or Afro - carribean ethnicity, decisions to screen should be individualised. AUA Guidelines, 2013.
- The risk of prostate cancer in these groups is far higher.

Causes

- Causes
- Cancer (Prostate cancer - adenocarcinoma)
- Infection: UTI, prostatitis
- Prostatic calculic
- Trauma to the prostate - catheterisation, flexible cystoscopy
- BPH - enlarged prostate

S. S. Goonewardene et al., *Basic Urological Management*,
https://doi.org/10.1007/978-3-319-98720-0_5

History

- UTIs, STIs.
- LUTS - storage (Frequency, urgency, nocturia) and voiding (weak stream, strain, hesitancy), post micturition (terminal dribbling).
- IPSS scoring.
- Erectile function (SHIM score) and continence.
- Abdominal pain - retention.
- Red flags: weight loss bony aches backache.
- Past urological history: stones, trauma, cancer.
- Family history of prostate cancer - having 1 relative affected doubles your risk.

Examination

- Abdomen: palpable masses in flanks (renal mass), flank tenderness/ iliac fossa tenderness (stones), SPC mass (bladder mass or retention).
- Review of extermal genitalia with a chaperone (epididymo-orchitis), review of external meatus for stenosis.
- DRE: size, consistency, firmness of prostate gland (prostate cancer, EAU Guidelines 2018), nodular prostate (BPH/ prostate cancer, post TURP) boggy tender prostate (prostatitis, abcess).

Investigations

- As per EAU and NICE Guidance
- Urine dip and culture
- Repeat PSA - elevated on 2 samples
- MRI pelvis prostate with contrast
- If MRI positive (PIRADS 4 or 5), for transperineal template biopsy of prostate
- Target biopsies of affected regions on MRI

Outcome

- Identify patient performance status, fitness for anaesthetic and surgery.
- Discuss imaging and biopsies results at Prostate MDT.
- Mapping meeting prior to target biopsies.
- Risk stratify patient into low intermediate or high risk. EAU Guidelines, 2018.

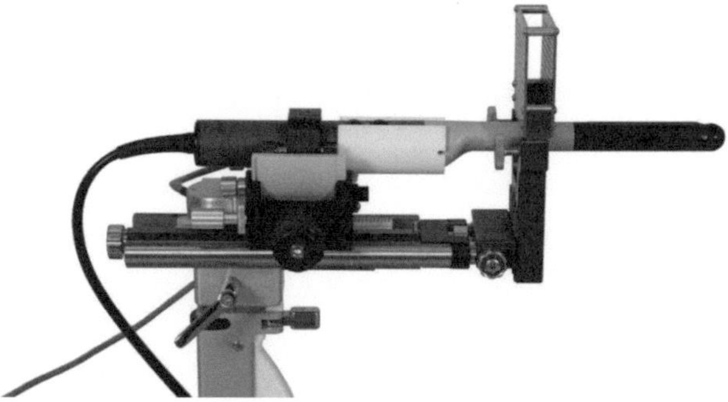

Fig. 5.1 Transperineal template biopsy probe and mount. It is imperative, everything is put together correctly and the probe is positioned correctly. If this is the case, the operation will be straightforward. If not, you do not know the sectors you are taking the biopsies from

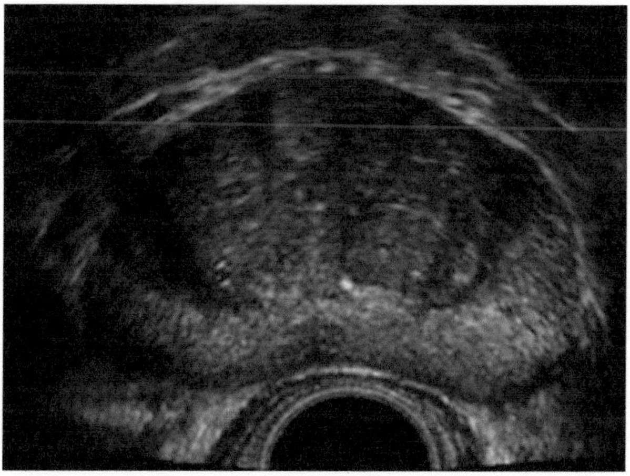

Fig. 5.2 Appearance of prostate via transrectal uss probe

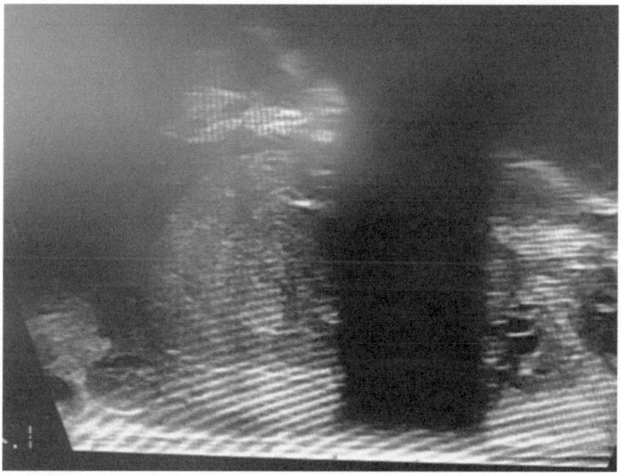

Fig. 5.3 A transrectal probe with air artefact on screen- take the probe out, re prep it and re-insert

Suggested Reading

AUA Guidelines, Early Detection of Prostate Cancer, 2015.
EAU Guidelines on Prostate Cancer, 2018.
NICE Guidance NG 2, 2008.

Diagnostic Pathway for Prostate Cancer

6

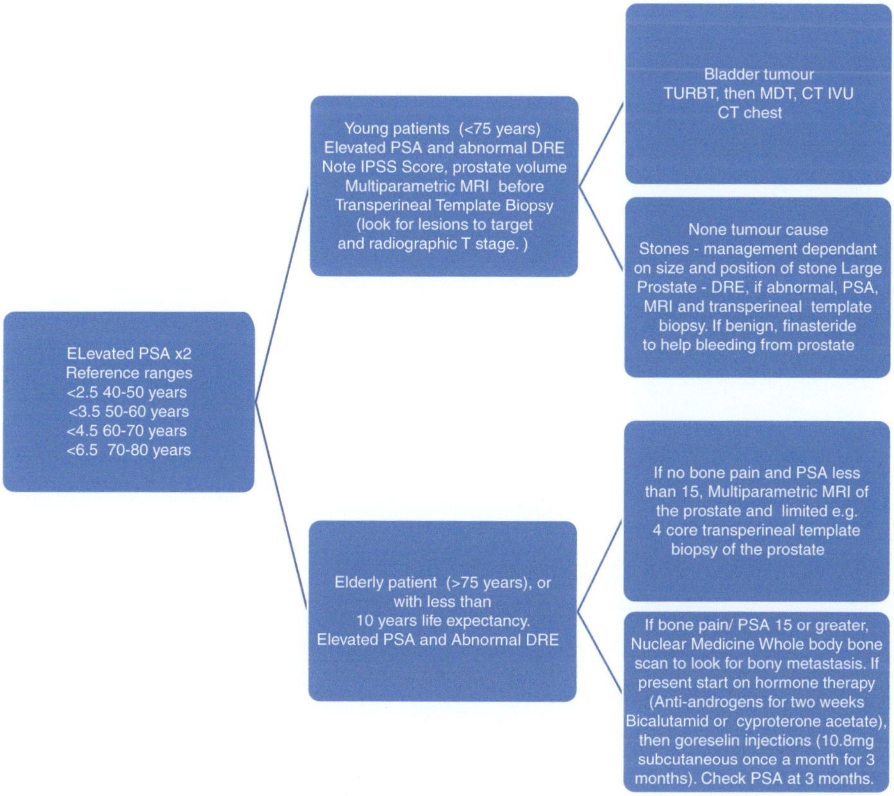

S. S. Goonewardene et al., *Basic Urological Management*,
https://doi.org/10.1007/978-3-319-98720-0_6

Suggested Reading

AUA Guidelines, Early Detection of Prostate Cancer, 2015.
EAU Guidelines on Prostate Cancer, 2018.
NICE Guidance NG 2, 2008.

7 Management Pathway for Prostate Cancer in Younger Patients

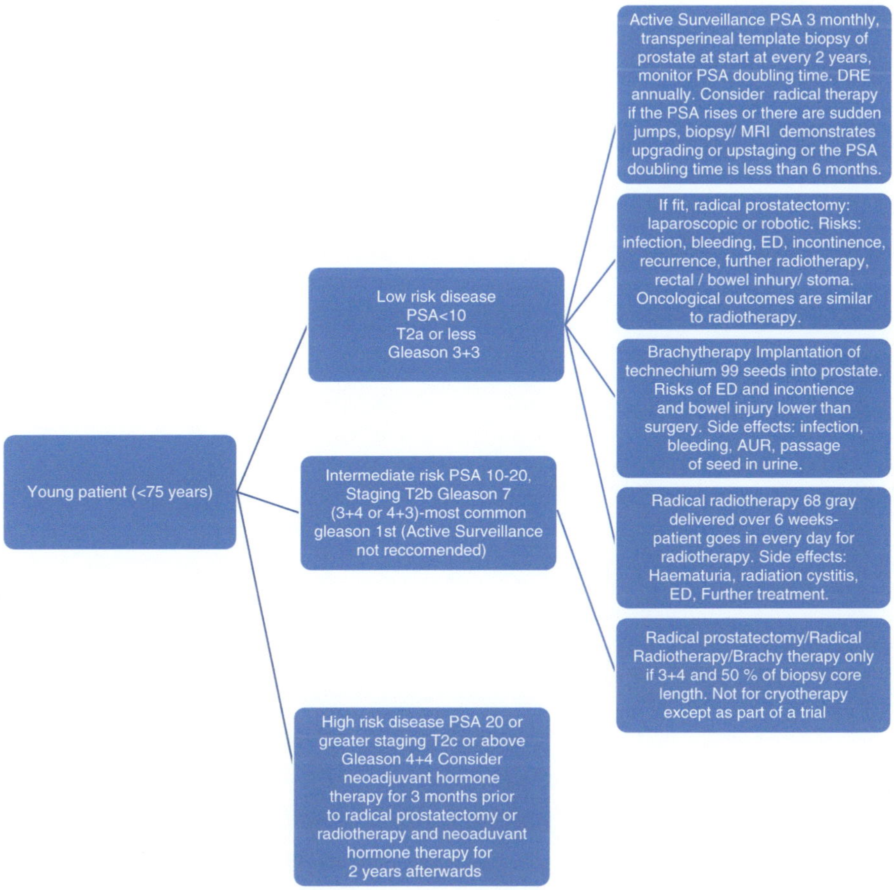

S. S. Goonewardene et al., *Basic Urological Management*,
https://doi.org/10.1007/978-3-319-98720-0_7

Suggested Reading

AUA Guidelines, Early Detection of Prostate Cancer, 2015.
EAU Guidelines on Prostate Cancer, 2018.
NICE Guidance NG 2, 2008.

Management Pathway for Older Patients with Prostate Cancer

8

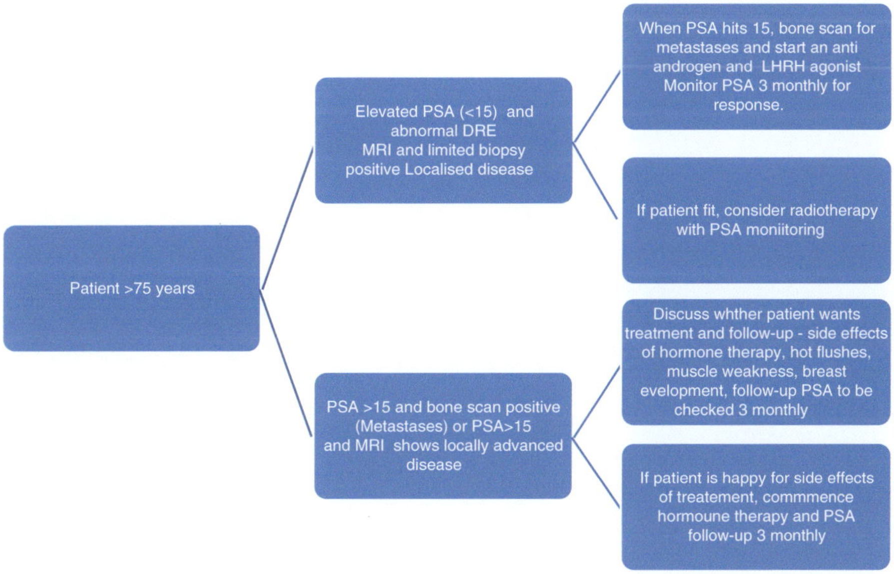

Suggested Reading

AUA Guidelines, Early Detection of Prostate Cancer, 2015.
EAU Guidelines on Prostate Cancer, 2018.
NICE Guidance NG 2, 2008.

S. S. Goonewardene et al., *Basic Urological Management*,
https://doi.org/10.1007/978-3-319-98720-0_8

Management of TRUS Biopsy Sepsis

9

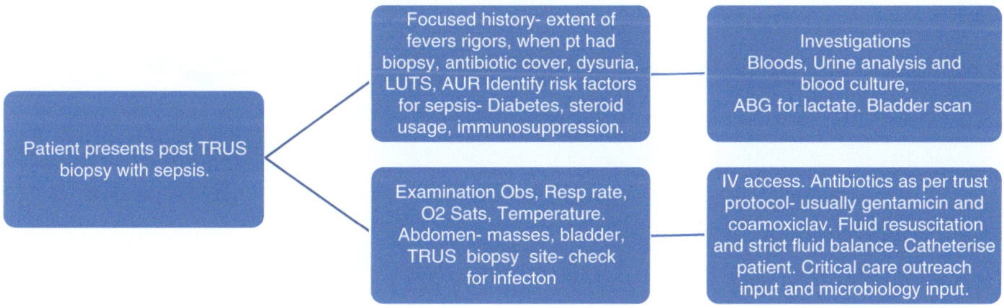

S. S. Goonewardene et al., *Basic Urological Management*,
https://doi.org/10.1007/978-3-319-98720-0_9

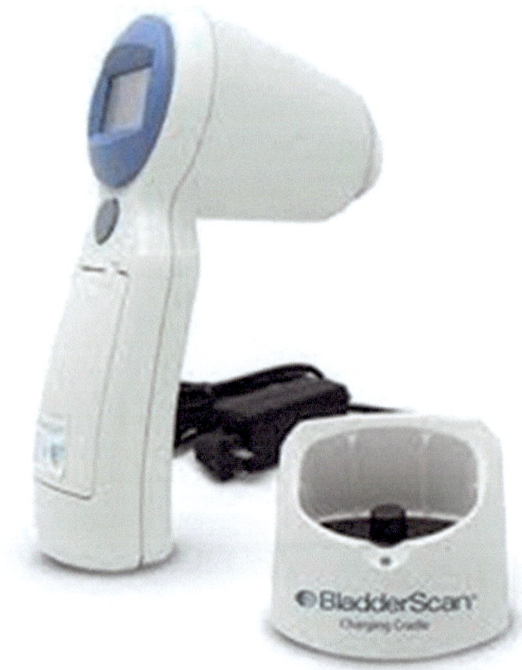

Fig. 9.1 A bladder scanner- a post void scan of < 200 ml is acceptable

Suggested Reading

Anderson E, Leahy O, Cheng AC, Grummet J. Risk factors for infection following prostate biopsy - a case control study. BMC Infect Dis. 2015;15:580.

Roth H, Millar JL, Cheng AC, Byrne A, Evans S, Grummet J. The state of TRUS biopsy sepsis: readmissions to Victorian hospitals with TRUS biopsy-related infection over 5 years. BJU Int. 2015;116(Suppl 3):49–53.

10 Haematospermia

Referral criteria

- As per NICE Guidelines on Cancer recognition.
- >40 years with no identifiable cause.
- Menof any age with signs and symptoms suggestive of prostate cancer (such as elevated PSA levels, suspicious findings on digital rectal examination).
- Signs or symptoms suggestive oftesticularor urological malignancies.
- >Ten episodes of haematospermia, with no identifiable cause found in primary care.
- Cysts or calculi of the prostate or seminal vesicles.
- Persistent haematospermia.

Causes

- Causes, Drake T et al, 2016.
- Cancer: Prostate cancer, epididymal, or testicular cancer.
- Infection: UTI/ STI, epididymo-orchitis, infection of seminal vesicles, Schistosoma haematobium and Trichomonas.
- Inflammation-Chronic or acuteprostatitis (chronic pelvic pain syndrome), urethritis.
- Stones: prostatic, bladder, ureteric calculi.
- Bleeding disorders or anticoagulation.
- Trauma to the urinary tract, post op, post TRUS biopsy, post brachytherapy.

S. S. Goonewardene et al., *Basic Urological Management*,
https://doi.org/10.1007/978-3-319-98720-0_10

History

- Ng Y 2013 et al.
- History: when, how often, STIs, UTIS, perineal pain, bleeding diathesis/anticoagulation, LUTs, malignant hypertension.
- Family history of prostate cancer or urological cancers.
- Recent instrumentation.
- Travel history: any recent foreign travel abroad-schistosoma/ TB.
- Past urological history: stones, trauma, cancer, prostatitis.

Examination

- BP
- SPC mass (bladder mass).
- Scrotal examination (penile lesions, palpate the vas-is it TB?), review of external urethral meatus-discharge (STI).
- Examine the testes and epidydimis (TB or tumour).
- DRE: size, consistency, firmness of prostate gland (prostate cancer), tenderness (prostatitis), seminal vesicles (usually none palpable, if palpable,? prostate cancer).

Investigations

- As Per NICE Guidance.
- Urine analysis and culture.
- First line investigations.
  - Flexible cystoscopy-if urine analysis negative.
  - CT IVU-look for a cause of haematuria that could be presenting as haematospermia.
- Urine cytology.
- STI screen if indicated at a GU clinic.
- PSA if abnormal DRE.
- If persistent haematuria, second line investigations: MRI and TRUS biopsy of prostate.

Outcome

- Treat the cause.
- Infection UTI/ STI screen -send off cultures, treat with antibiotics according to hospital policy.
- Chronic or acute prostatitis (chronic pelvic pain syndrome) - As per NICE guideline, Ciprofloxacin 500 mg PO BD, with Tamsulosin 0.4 mg PO OD and an NSAID.
- Prostate cancer- check 2 PSAs, MRI prostate or bone scan as appropriate, then Prostate MDT follow-up.
- Trauma to the urinary tract-treat according to severity and site of trauma- conservative (renal trauma grades 1-4 if HD stable), vs suirgical management (renal truama grade 5) - see trauma chapters.
- Exotic infections such as *Schistosoma haematobium* and *Trichomonas* spp-infectious diseases review.

Suggested Reading

Drake T, Hanna L, Davies M. Haematospermia (Practice). BMJ. 2016;355:i5124.
Ng Y, Seeley J, Smith G. Haematospermia as a presenting symptom: outcomes of investigation in 300 men. Surgeon. 2013;11(1):35–8.
NICE Clinical Knowledge Summary on Haematospermia.

11 Diagnostic and Management Pathway for Haematospermia

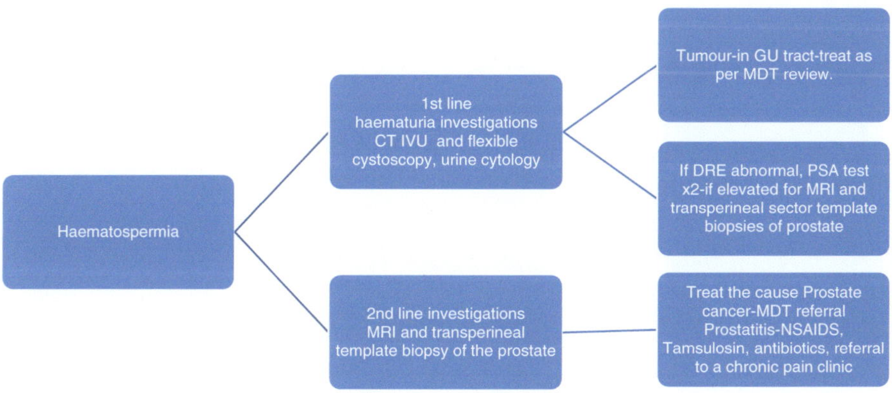

Suggested Reading

Drake T, Hanna L, Davies M. Haematospermia (Practice). BMJ. 2016;355:i5124.

Ng Y, Seeley J, Smith G. Haematospermia as a presenting symptom: outcomes of investigation in 300 men. Surgeon. 2013;11(1):35–8.

NICE Clinical Knowledge Summary on Haematospermia.

S. S. Goonewardene et al., *Basic Urological Management*,
https://doi.org/10.1007/978-3-319-98720-0_11

12 Lower Urinary Tract Symptoms

Referral criteria

- As per NICE Guidance CG 12, 2015.
- LUTS complicated by recurrent or persistent urinary tract infection, retention, renal impairment that is suspected to be caused by lower urinary tract dysfunction, or suspected urological cancer.
- Men with stress urinary incontinence.
- Bothersome LUTS that have not responded to conservative management or drug treatment.
- Patients with failed medical therapy requiring surgical treatment options or catheterisation (ISC, SPC or urethral).

Causes

- Anatomical obstruction: Benign prostatic hyperplasia (BPH), urethral stricture, prostate cancer.
- Detrusor muscle weakness and/or instability, OAB.
- Infection: Urinary Tract Infection (UTI)/STI, prostatitis.
- Inflammation: chronic prostatitis, urethritis.
- Stones-bladder or ureteric stones.
- Cancer: prostate or bladder cancer, urethral cancer.
- Neurological disease, e.g. multiple sclerosis, spinal cord injury, cauda equina syndrome.

S. S. Goonewardene et al., *Basic Urological Management*,
https://doi.org/10.1007/978-3-319-98720-0_12

History

- Take a Focused history, AUA Guidance on BPH, 2014.
- History: IPSS score, storage symptoms: frequency, urgency, nocturia, voiding symptoms: weak strain, stream, hesitancy, terminal dribbling, quality of life.
- STIs, UTIS, haematuria (visible/none visible).
- Waking up wet at night (chronic retention-high pressure-needs a catheter immediately).
- Fevers/rigors (sepsis).
- Prior therapy or investigations-any under urology.
- Past urological history: catheters, AUR, prostate cancer, urological procedures.

Examination

- BP.
- Abdomen: palpable masses in flanks (renal mass), flank tenderness (stones), SPC mass (bladder mass or retention).
- Scrotal examination-evidence of epididymoorchitis, testicular or penile masses, review of external urethral meatus-size.
- Catheters-size, type (urethral/ SPC/ LTC?), colour of urine draining, debris/clots.
- DRE: size, consistency, firmness of prostate gland.

Investigations

- As per EAU Guidance, 2018.
- Urine analysis and culture.
- Flow rate including voided volume (difficult to interpret if less than 100 mls). Expect the curve of BPH on flow rate.
- Post void scan (less than 200 mls is acceptable).
- Renal function, if abnormal, USS KUB (review for bilateral hydronephrosis, if present or if renal function deranged, catheterise).

Outcome

- Speakmann (2015), Oelke (2015)
- If BPH: Conservative management.
  - Cut out caffeine and diuretics.
  - Urethral sump milking (squeezing last few drops out of the urethra).
  - Bladder re-training.
- Medical management: tamsulosin, finasteride or combination therapy with an anticholinergic or antimuscarinic.
- Surgical management: TURP or LTC/ISC if patient not keen on operation.
- If urethral stricture
  - Flattened trace on flowrate -book for Flexible cystoscopy/ urethrogram.
  - Book for Rigid cystoscopy +/- urethral dilation or optical urethrtomy.

Suggested Reading

AUA Guidance on Management of BPH, 2014

EAU Guidelines on None Neurogenic Male LUTS, 2018.

NICE Guidance CG 67 on Male LUTS, 2015

Oelke M, Becher K, Castro-Diaz D, Chartier-Kastler E, Kirby M, Wagg A, Wehling M. Appropriateness of oral drugs for long-term treatment of lower urinary tract symptoms in older persons: results of a systematic literature review and international consensus validation process (LUTS-FORTA 2014). Age Ageing. 2015;44(5):745–55.

Speakman M, Kirby R, Doyle S, Ioannou C. Burden of male lower urinary tract symptoms (LUTS) suggestive of benign prostatic hyperplasia (BPH) - focus on the UK. BJU Int. 2015;115(4):508–19.

13 Diagnostic Pathway for LUTS

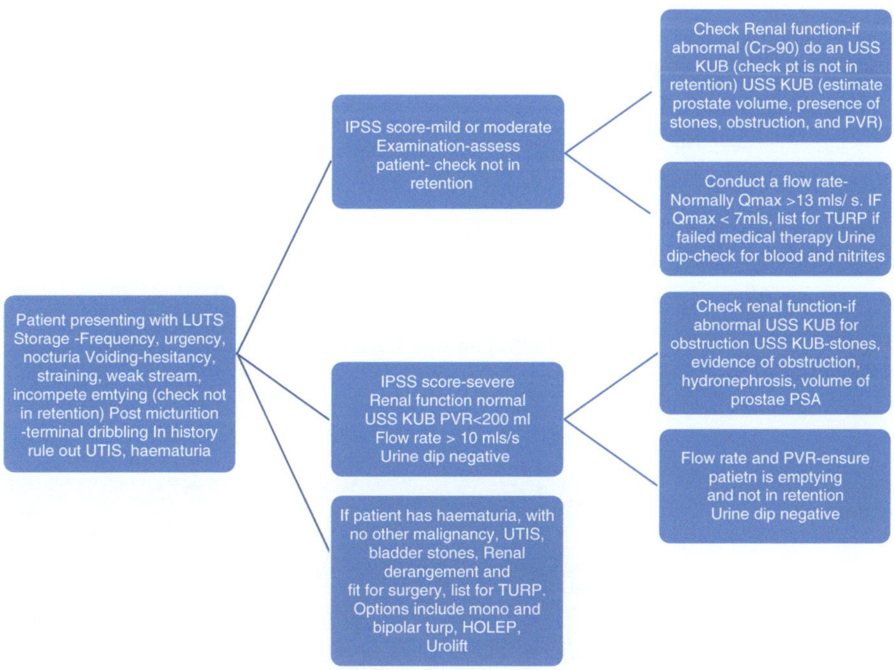

S. S. Goonewardene et al., *Basic Urological Management*,
https://doi.org/10.1007/978-3-319-98720-0_13

Fig. 13.1 MRI demonstrating large prostate with prostate cancer, protruding into bladder

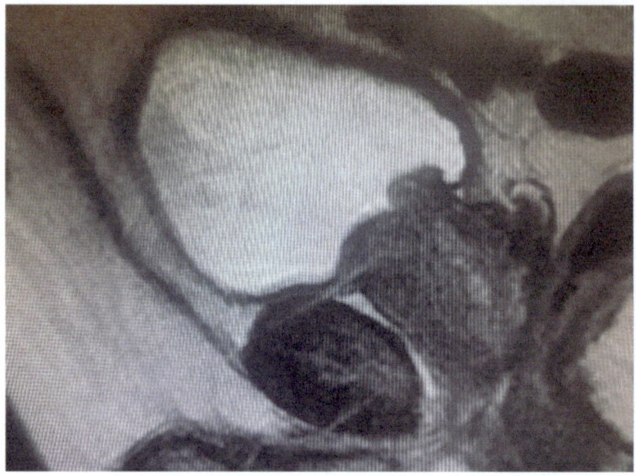

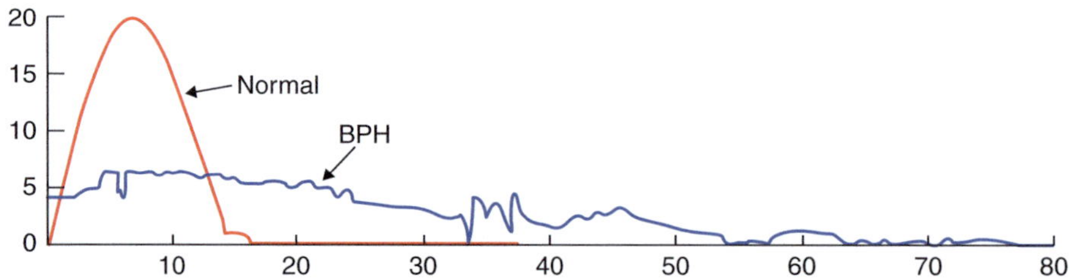

Fig. 13.2 Demonstrating normal and BPH flow rate. If a urethral stricture is present, you will see a flat line

Fig. 13.3 BPH on cystoscopy

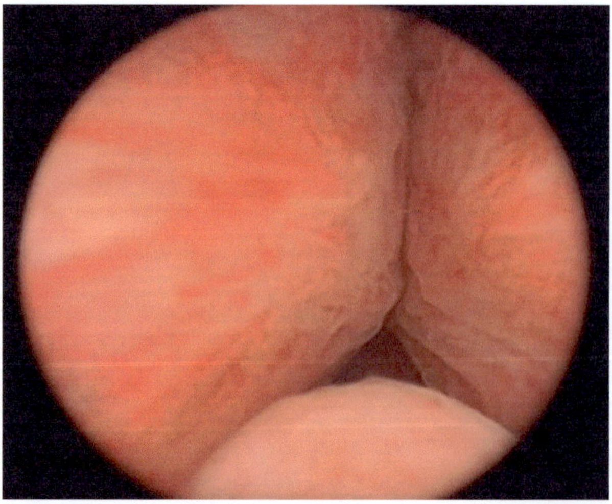

Suggested Reading

AUA Guidance on Management of BPH, 2014

EAU Guidelines on None Neurogenic Male LUTS, 2018

NICE Guidance CG 67 on Male LUTS, 2015

Oelke M, Becher K, Castro-Diaz D, Chartier-Kastler E, Kirby M, Wagg A, Wehling M. Appropriateness of oral drugs for long-term treatment of lower urinary tract symptoms in older persons: results of a systematic literature review and international consensus validation process (LUTS-FORTA 2014). Age Ageing. 2015;44(5):745–55.

Speakman M, Kirby R, Doyle S, Ioannou C. Burden of male lower urinary tract symptoms (LUTS) suggestive of benign prostatic hyperplasia (BPH) - focus on the UK. BJU Int. 2015;115(4):508–19.

Management Pathway for LUTS-Benign Prostatic Enlargement

14

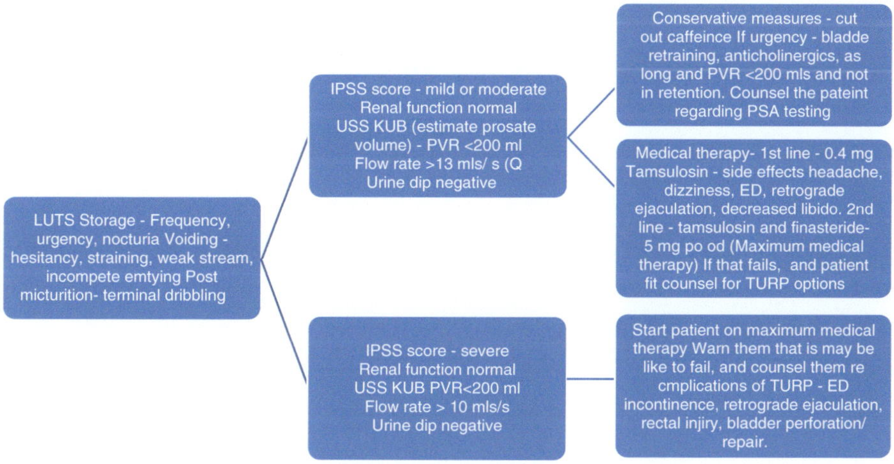

Suggested Reading

AUA Guidance on Management of BPH, 2014

EAU Guidelines on None Neurogenic Male LUTS, 2018.

NICE Guidance CG 67 on Male LUTS, 2015

Oelke M, Becher K, Castro-Diaz D, Chartier-Kastler E, Kirby M, Wagg A, Wehling M. Appropriateness of oral drugs for long-term treatment of lower urinary tract symptoms in older persons: results of a systematic literature review and international consensus validation process (LUTS-FORTA 2014). Age Ageing. 2015;44(5):745–55.

Speakman M, Kirby R, Doyle S, Ioannou C. Burden of male lower urinary tract symptoms (LUTS) suggestive of benign prostatic hyperplasia (BPH) - focus on the UK. BJU Int. 2015;115(4):508–19.

S. S. Goonewardene et al., *Basic Urological Management*,
https://doi.org/10.1007/978-3-319-98720-0_14

15 Acute Urinary Retention

Definition

- Acute presentation to A+E.
- Pain and inability to pass urine, despite desire to do so.
- Pain in suprapubic region.
- Pain relieved by catheterisation.
- (Cathcart et al)
- Usually > 600-800mls

Causes

- NICE Evidence Summary on Acute Urinary Retention.
- Anatomical causes: Benign prostatic hyperplasia (BPH) with obstruction, Prostate cancer and enlarged prostate, urethral stricture.
- Functional causes: Detrusor muscle weakness and/or instability.
- Neuropathic causes: Spinal injury, spinal column compromise, MS.
- Infectious causes: Urinary Tract Infection (UTI)/ Prostatic abcess/ Chronic prostatitis.
- Clot retention (bleeding from urinary tract, cancer cause)
- Pelvic causes: prolapse, pelvic masses, bladder cancer.
- Medical causes, consiptation, diabetes.
- Post op - instrumentation, cystoscopy, TRUS biopsy, hernia surgery, radical pelvic surgery, post GA.

History

- Catherise patient 1st - monitor residual. Note whether they are on anticoagulants or have had lower abodminal surgery, in case of difficult catheter and SPC requirement.
- History: IPSS score, storage symptoms: frequency, urgency, nocturia, voiding symptoms straining: weak strain, stream, hesitancy, terminal dribbling,
- STIs, UTIS, haematuria - if any haematuria - patient not for SPC (if cancer you can convert a localised tumour to an advanced one).
- Prior therapy, investigations. past history of retention.
- Past urological history: catheters, AUR, prostate cancer.
- As per Kirby et al.

S. S. Goonewardene et al., *Basic Urological Management*,
https://doi.org/10.1007/978-3-319-98720-0_15

Examination

- Monitor observations - if septic assess and treat cause.
- Abdomen: palpable masses in flanks (renal mass), flank tenderness (stones, pyelonephritis), SPC mass (bladder mass or retention)
- Scrotal examination, testis and epididymis - scrotal infection.
- Review of external urethral meatus - any discharge.
- DRE: size, consistency, firmness of prostate gland, tenderness (abcess, prostatitis).

Investigations

- Catheterise, IV antibiotics, one shot gentamicin usually.
- If septic, at least a 7 day course.
- Decompression may result in haematuria.
- Urine culture - once cultures are back, treat according to sensitivities - micro should be able to give a general indication within 24 hrs.
- Residual volume: if less than 600 mls, discharge home with OPA for TWOCK.
- If > 600 mls admit and monitor for diuresis.
- Lying and standing BP
- Renal function and USS KUB
- (EAU Guidelines on Male LUTS, 2018.)

Outcome

- Treat the cause
- If HPCR - TURP or LTC
- If AUR and PVR <800 mls, start tamsulosin 0.4 mg po od (works within 48 hours) and for TWOCK at later date. If TWOC failed, for TURP.
- If AUR and PVR > 800mls, for TURP or LTC/ ISC.

Suggested Reading

Cathcart P, van der Meulen J, Armitage J, et al. Incidence of primary and recurrent acute urinary retention between 1998 and 2003 in England. J Urol. 2006;176(1):200–4.

Fitzpatrick JM, Kirby RS. Management of acute urinary retention. BJU Int. 2006;97(Suppl 2):16–20.

Gratzke C, Bachmann A, Descazeaud A, Drake MJ, Madersbacher S, Mamoulakis C, Oelke M, Tikkinen KAO, Gravas S. EAU guidelines on the assessment of non-neurogenic male lower urinary tract symptoms including benign prostatic obstruction. Eur Urol. 2015;67(6):1099–109.

NICE Evidence Summary on Acute Urinary Retention. 2018.

16 Diagnostic Pathway for Acute Urinary Retention

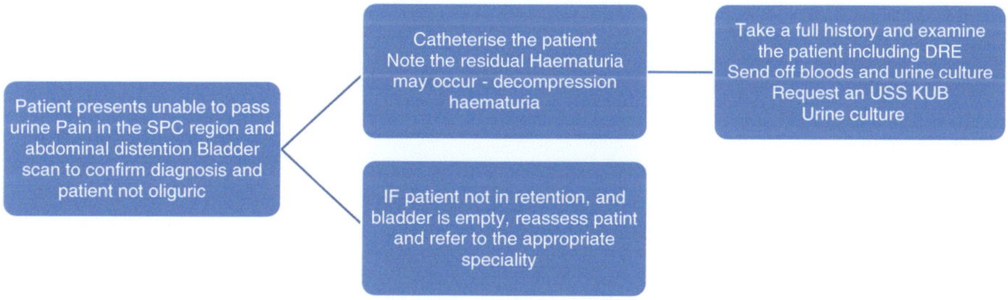

Suggested Reading

Cathcart P, van der Meulen J, Armitage J, et al. Incidence of primary and recurrent acute urinary retention between 1998 and 2003 in England. J Urol. 2006;176(1):200–4.

Fitzpatrick JM, Kirby RS. Management of acute urinary retention. BJU Int. 2006;97(Suppl 2):16–20.

Gratzke C, Bachmann A, Descazeaud A, Drake MJ, Madersbacher S, Mamoulakis C, Oelke M, Tikkinen KAO, Gravas S. EAU guidelines on the assessment of non-neurogenic male lower urinary tract symptoms including benign prostatic obstruction. Eur Urol. 2015;67(6):1099–109.

NICE Evidence Summary on Acute Urinary Retention. 2018.

S. S. Goonewardene et al., *Basic Urological Management*,
https://doi.org/10.1007/978-3-319-98720-0_16

17 Management Pathway for Acute Urinary Retention

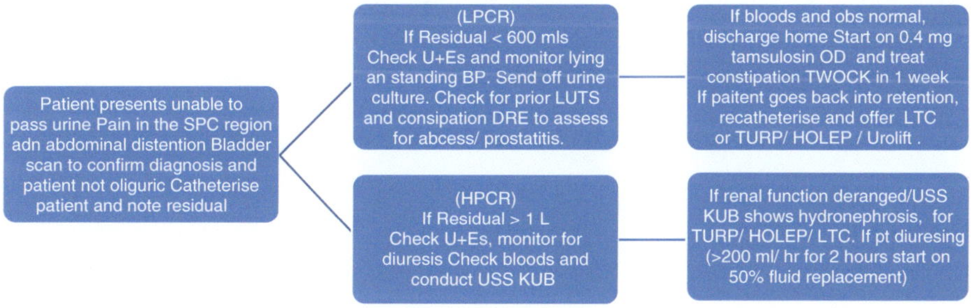

Suggested Reading

Oelke M, Bachmann A, Descazeaud A, Emberton M, Gravas S, Michel MC, N'dow J, Nordling J, de la Rosette JJ. EAU guidelines on the treatment and follow-up of non-neurogenic male lower urinary tract symptoms including benign prostatic obstruction. Eur Urol. 2013;64(1):118–40.

Oelke M, Burger M, Castro-Diaz D, Chartier-Kastler E, Jimènez Cidre MA, McNicholas T, Radziszewski P, Kirby M. Diagnosis and medical treatment of lower urinary tract symptoms in adult men: applying specialist guidelines in clinical practice. BJU Int. 2012;110(5):710–8.

S. S. Goonewardene et al., *Basic Urological Management*,
https://doi.org/10.1007/978-3-319-98720-0_17

18 Difficult Catheters

Definition

- A catheter which does not pass smoothly and easily up the urethra (meatal, bulbourethra, prostatic and membranous urethra) into the bladder.
- Do not force catheter up the urethra - it is very easy to traumatise this region, redering the patient susceptible to urethral strictures and surgery for life.
- If a catheter is forced on an introducer, this can cause bleeding requiring emergency surgery.
- Gentle and smooth insertion is the best way forward. Prentiss et al, 1969.

Causes

- Causes of AUR.
- Benign prostatic hyperplasia (BPH) with obstruction/prostate cancer.
- Bladder stone / prostatic or urethral calculi.
- Chronic prostatitis.
- Urethral stricture, urethral flap, prior urethroplasty.
- TCC, bladder or urethra.
- Iatrogenic, post TRUS biopsy, post instrumentation.

S. S. Goonewardene et al., *Basic Urological Management*,
https://doi.org/10.1007/978-3-319-98720-0_18

Urethral catheterisation

- Keep the pt NBM and check clotting (note anticoagulants and revesal agents)
- Assess the abdomen for lower abdominal scars - enquire about haematuria (not for SPC, only for flexible cystoscopy guided catheter).
- Palpate for a palpable bladder (acute retention, volume > 600 mls needed for SPC to be safe).
- If prior attempts have been made, localise where the problem is - meatus, bulbourethra or prostate.
- Have one go at catheterisation with a LTC - 16 fr, LTC 18 fr.
- If you feel resistance don't push move onto the next step (below)
- (Willette et al 2012).

Coude tip catheters

- Catheters with a curved tip.
- Also known as Tiemanns tip.
- Purpose of curve - to negotiate urethral flaps, strictures or large prostates.
- Hold the catheter upright and glide it along the urethra - a 16 fr first.
- If you encounter obstruction, don't push. - you could traumatize the urethra.

Flexible cystoscopy guided catheter

- Indication - failure of urethral catheter using either standard urethral catheters or Coude tip catheters.
- Place to do it - theatre anaesthetic room - under LA.
- Equipment: flexible cystoscopy, light source, monitor, giving set, Normal saline 500 ml bag, sensor guidewire (hydrophilic guidewire), venflon.
- Via aseptic technique, connect the light source to the flexible cystoscopy. Connect the giving set to the fluid and to the cystoscope.
- Fill the chamber and get rid of air bubbles. Prep and drape the area, instill the LA into the urethra.
- Pass the flexible cystoscopy into the bladder, then pass the guidewire, and railroad the catheter over it using the venflon.
- Monitor the residual volume post procedure.
- (Wagner et al, Abbott et al,)

Supra-pubic catheter

- Assess the patient for haematuria. If present, they may have a TCC bladder - do not do an SPC.
- If there are any lower midline scars, the patient will need an open cystoscopy instead, under GA.
- Check the clotting. Make sure the patient is appropriately consented - bowel perforation, vascular damage, open surgical repair.
- Get the kit ready first (seldinger technique): 2% lidocaine with adrenaline -10 mls drawn up. Spinal needle ready. Guidewire - with a soft tip. Dilator and trochar ready.
- Infiltrate the LA in a bleb under the skin 1-2 cm above the symphisis pubis in the midline, then down to the bladder and aspirate. Do not insert the SPC unless urine is aspriated. Attach the syringe to the spinal needle and re-insert over the LA infiltration site., aspirate as you go down. You are in the bladder if you can aspirate 10 mls of urine.
- Remove the syringe and pass the guidewire (soft tip 1st) into the bladder.
- Insert dilator and trochar over that once skin has been incised.
- Remove the dilator and guidewire, put a tube of instillagel down the trochar (gives you more time) and insert the 16 fr catheter that came with the set.
- (Ghaffary et al)

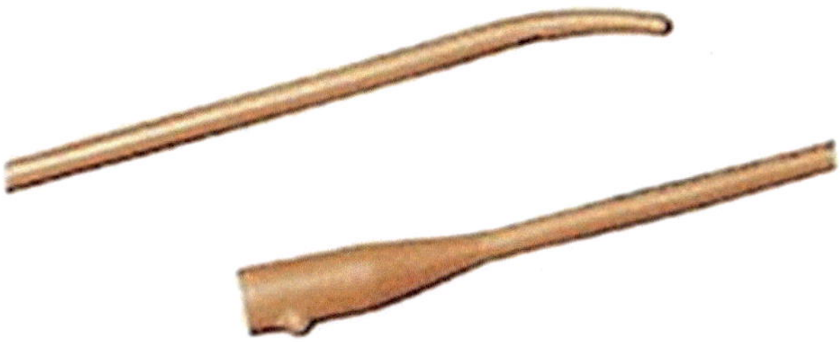

Fig. 18.1 A Coude tip catheter

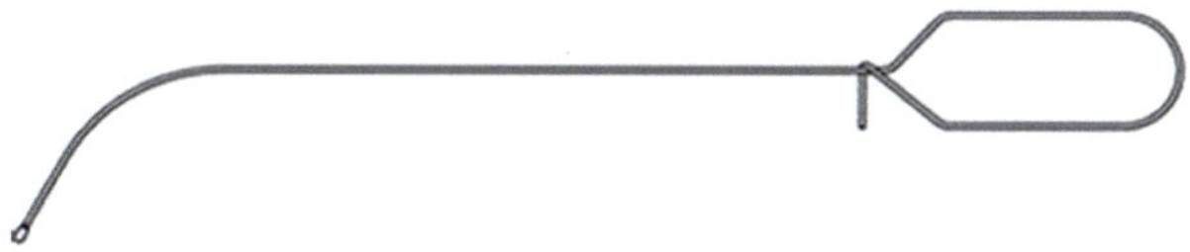

Fig. 18.2 An Introducer- usually passed down a catheter and used to insert the catheter urethrally. The curve can be used to slide the tip over the side of the bladder

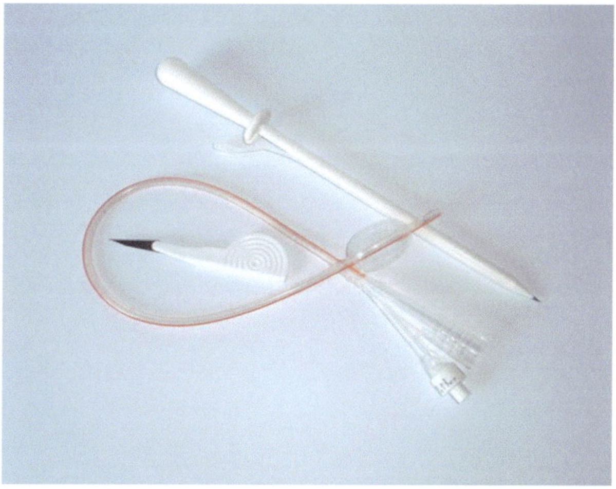

Fig. 18.3 Supra-pubic catheter set

Suggested Reading

Abbott JE, Heinemann A, Badalament R, Davalos JG. A clever technique for placement of a urinary catheter over a wire. Urol Ann. 2015;7(3):367–70.

Ghaffary C, Yohannes A, Villanueva C, Leslie SW. A practical approach to difficult urinary catheterizations. Curr Urol Rep. 2013;14(6):565–79.

Prentiss RJ, Mullenix RB, Feeney MJ, Howe GE, Steel JF, Cole JW, Flynn VJ, Walther AB, Sorensen MB. The catheter. How to use and when not to use. Calif Med. 1969;111(4):265–71.

Tadtayev S, Mazaris E. Difficult urethral catheterisation made easy: validation and the new application of the established technique. Ann R Coll Surg Engl. 2013;95(4):300.

Wagner KR, Bird ET, Coffield KS. Urinary catheterization: a paradigm shift in difficult urinary catheterization. Curr Urol Rep. 2016;17(11):82.

Willette PA, Coffield S. Current trends in the management of difficult urinary catheterizations. West J Emerg Med. 2012;13(6):472–8.

Management Pathway for Difficult Catheters

19

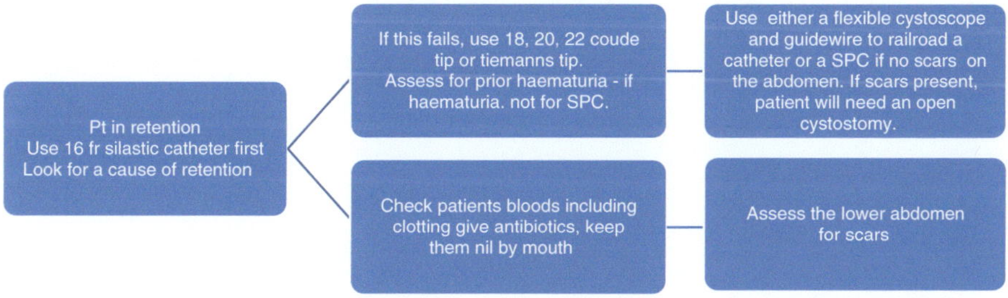

Suggested Reading

Prentiss RJ, Mullenix RB, Feeney MJ, Howe GE, Steel JF, Cole JW, Flynn VJ, Walther AB, Sorensen MB. The catheter. How to use and when not to use. Calif Med. 1969;111(4):265–71.

Tadtayev S, Mazaris E. Difficult urethral catheterisation made easy: validation and the new application of the established technique. Ann R Coll Surg Engl. 2013;95(4):300.

Wagner KR, Bird ET, Coffield KS. Urinary catheterization: a paradigm shift in difficult urinary catheterization. Curr Urol Rep. 2016;17(11):82.

Willette PA, Coffield S. Current trends in the management of difficult urinary catheterizations. West J Emerg Med. 2012;13(6):472–8.

S. S. Goonewardene et al., *Basic Urological Management*,
https://doi.org/10.1007/978-3-319-98720-0_19

20 Chronic Retention

Definition

- Chronic presentation, very often to OPA.
- Despite voiding, patient still has full bladder, which is painless.
- Patients often deny problems.
- A very small volume would be passed (overflow) usually as dribbling.
- No pain, with a palpable bladder.
- Patient may decribe difficulty voiding and waking up wet at night.
- Volume greater than 800 ml.
- (Negro et al)

Causes

- Benign prostatic hyperplasia (BPH) with obstruction.
- Prostate cancer.
- Detrusor muscle weakness and/or instability.
- Neuropathic bladder.
- Chronic prostatitis.
- Urethral/meatal stricture or phimosis stricture.
- (Chapple et al. 2013)

History

- As per NICE Guidance
- Catherise patient 1st. Patient will very often wake up wet at night.
- History: IPSS score, voiding: frequency, urgency, nocturia, straining: weak strain, stream, hesitancy, terminal dribbling, STIs, UTIS.
- Prior therapy, investigations. past history of retention, therapy.
- Past urological history: catheters, AUR, prostate cancer.

S. S. Goonewardene et al., *Basic Urological Management*,
https://doi.org/10.1007/978-3-319-98720-0_20

Suggested Reading

Negro CL, Muir GH. Chronic urinary retention in men: how we define it, and how does it affect treatment outcome. BJU Int. 2012;110(11):1590–4.

NICE Guidelines CG 97, Lower urinary tract symptoms in men: management. 2015

Osman NI, Chapple CR. Chronic urinary retention in men: how we define it, and how does it affect treatment outcome. BJU Int. 2013;111(4):E138–9.

21 Diagnostic Pathway for Chronic Retention

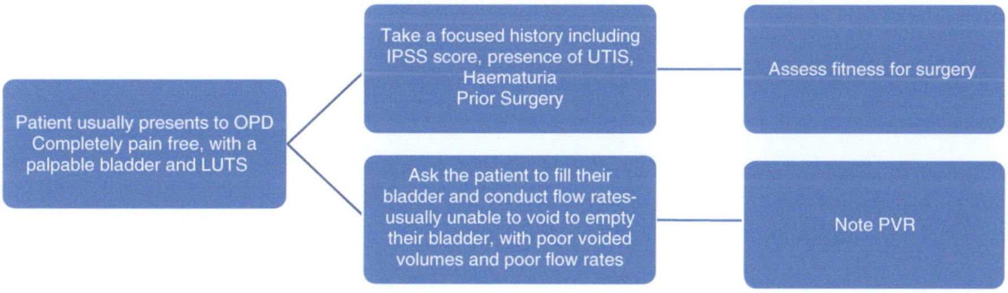

Suggested Reading

Negro CL, Muir GH. Chronic urinary retention in men: how we define it, and how does it affect treatment outcome. BJU Int. 2012;110(11):1590–4.

NICE Guidelines CG 97. Lower urinary tract symptoms in men: management. 2015.

Osman NI, Chapple CR. Chronic urinary retention in men: how we define it, and how does it affect treatment outcome. BJU Int. 2013;111(4):E138–9.

S. S. Goonewardene et al., *Basic Urological Management*,
https://doi.org/10.1007/978-3-319-98720-0_21

Management Pathway for Chronic Retention

22

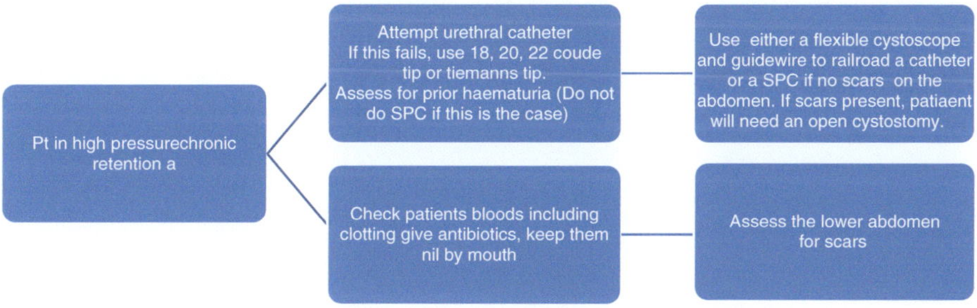

Suggested Reading

Negro CL, Muir GH. Chronic urinary retention in men: how we define it, and how does it affect treatment outcome. BJU Int. 2012;110(11):1590–4.

NICE Guidelines CG 97. Lower urinary tract symptoms in men: management. 2015.

Osman NI, Chapple CR. Chronic urinary retention in men: how we define it, and how does it affect treatment outcome. BJU Int. 2013;111(4):E138–9.

S. S. Goonewardene et al., *Basic Urological Management*,
https://doi.org/10.1007/978-3-319-98720-0_22

Metastatic Spinal Cord Compression 23

Definition

- Mobility threatening (Nair et al)
- Loss of innervation from the lumbar plexus (nerve roots) of the spinal canal below the termination (conus medullaris) of the spinal cord.
- Lower motor neurone lesion.
- First sign is acute urinary retention - if this is diagnosed, always check sensation (saddle anaesthesiae) and anal tone.
- Once catheterised, MRI immediately.

Causes

- As per NICE Guidance
- Tumour: compression from metastatic prostate cancer - maybe in multiple vertebrae.
- Trauma - fracture of vertebral bodies, destabilisation of the spinal column and compression.
- Spinal canal stenosis, lumbar disc protrusion.
- Infection, bleeding.
- Demyelinating conditions - MS.
- AV Malformation.

History

- History: IPSS score, LUTS. Back pain. UTIS. Mobility issues.
- Saddle anaesthesiae, sciatic pain.
- AUR - if so for how long - acute on chronic? Any problems or recurrent episodes of retention before?
- History of tumour, trauma, neuropathy (motor or sensory), sexual dysfunction.
- Try to localise spinal and neuropathic level - sensory and motor issues.
- Mobility - extent and duration of problems - gait disturbance.
- (Sun et al)

S. S. Goonewardene et al., *Basic Urological Management*,
https://doi.org/10.1007/978-3-319-98720-0_23

Examination

- Full neurological exam - upper and lower limbs and cranial nerves - reduced reflexes
- Abdomen: palpable masses in flanks (renal mass/ hydronephrosis), flank tenderness (stones), SPC mass (bladder)
- Scrotal examination, review of external urethral meatus.
- DRE: anal tone, sensation, saddle anaesthesiae.
- Keep on bed rest.
- (Sun et al)

Investigations

- MRI spine - delineate level and extent of compression - assess the vertebrae above and below
- Bed rest and TEDS (neurosurgeons may request flowtrons/ heparin if for surgery). If a patient is on bed rest - increased risk of DVT formation.
- Dexamethosone 8 mg PO BD and a PPI
- Bloods including clotting and group & save
- Keep pt NBM in case of surgery.

Outcome

- Inform oncology and neurosurgeons of the MRI result.
- If the vertebrae above and below the compression are free of disease and the patient is fit, neurosurgery will decompress the spinal cord and plate this.
- If there is disease present above and below, then referral to radiation oncology is needed, where the patient will go for radiation therapy everyday for one week.
- Keep patient on bed rest with TEDS.
- Once decompressed/ treated with radiation therapy, start rehabilitaiton and make sure the cause is treated.

Suggested Reading

Brooks FM, Ghatahora A, Brooks MC, Warren H, Price L, Brahmabhatt P, De Vauvert S, John C, Farnworth E, Sulaiman E, Ahuja S. Management of metastatic spinal cord compression: awareness of NICE guidance. Eur J Orthop Surg Traumatol. 2014;24(Suppl 1):S255–9.

Nair C, Panikkar S, Ray A. How not to miss metastatic spinal cord compression. Br J Gen Pract. 2014;64(626):e596–8.

Savage P, Sharkey R, Kua T, Schofield L, Richardson D, Panchmatia N, Papanastasopoulos P, Williams M, Falconer A, Power D, Arnold F, Ulbricht C. Malignant spinal cord compression: NICE guidance, improvements and challenges. QJM. 2014;107(4):277–82.

Sun JC, Xu T, Chen KF, Qian W, Liu K, Shi JG, Yuan W, Jia LS. Assessment of cauda equina syndrome progression pattern to improve diagnosis. Spine (Phila Pa 1976). 2014;39(7):596–602.

24 Diagnostic Pathway for Metastatic Spinal Cord Compression

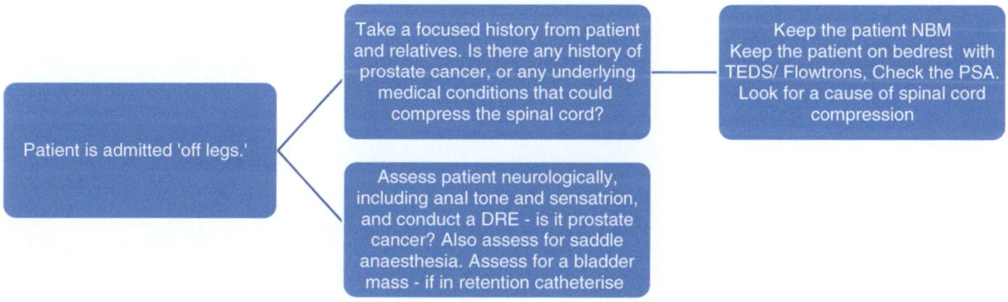

S. S. Goonewardene et al., *Basic Urological Management*,
https://doi.org/10.1007/978-3-319-98720-0_24

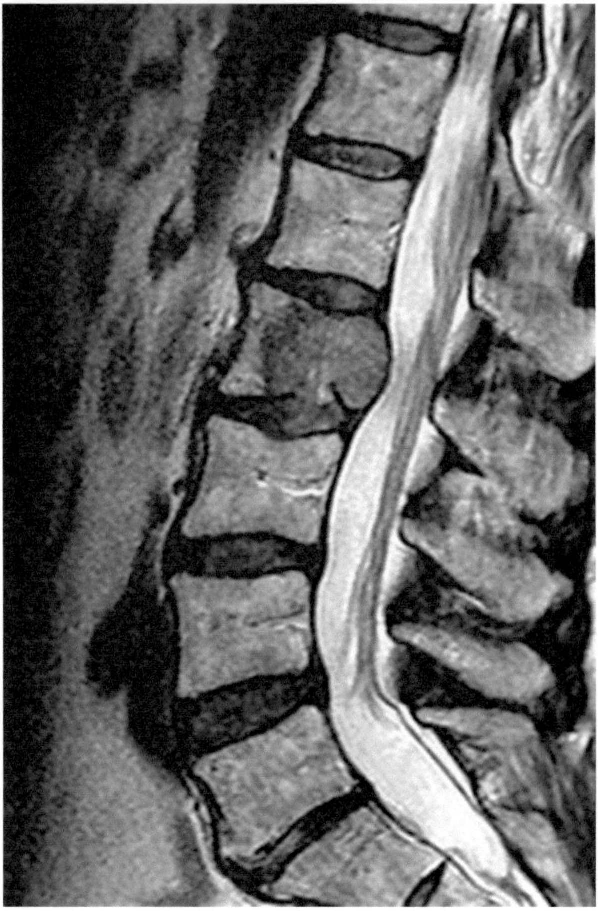

Fig. 24.1 MRI demonstrating metastatic spinal cord compression

Suggested Reading

Nair C, Panikkar S, Ray A. How not to miss metastatic spinal cord compression. Br J Gen Pract. 2014;64(626):e596–8.

Savage P, Sharkey R, Kua T, Schofield L, Richardson D, Panchmatia N, Papanastasopoulos P, Williams M, Falconer A, Power D, Arnold F, Ulbricht C. Malignant spinal cord compression: NICE guidance, improvements and challenges. QJM. 2014;107(4):277–82.

Sun JC, Xu T, Chen KF, Qian W, Liu K, Shi JG, Yuan W, Jia LS. Assessment of cauda equina syndrome progression pattern to improve diagnosis. Spine (Phila Pa 1976). 2014;39(7):596–602.

25 Management Pathway for Metstatic Spinal Cord Compression

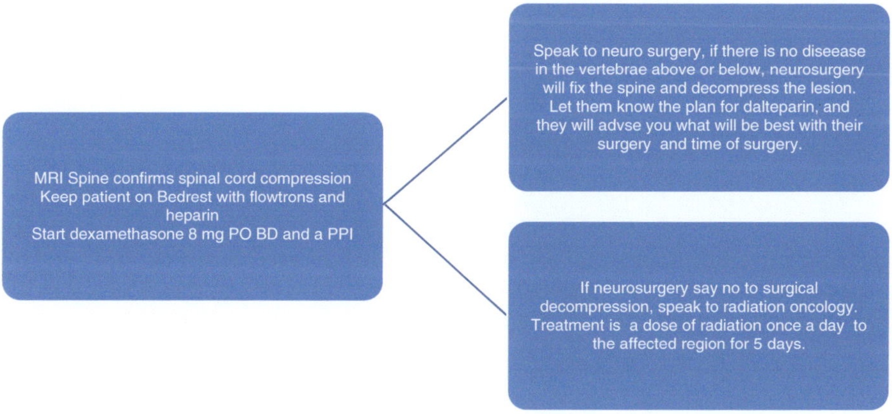

Suggested Reading

Brooks FM, Ghatahora A, Brooks MC, Warren H, Price L, Brahmabhatt P, De Vauvert S, John C, Farnworth E, Sulaiman E, Ahuja S. Management of metastatic spinal cord compression: awareness of NICE guidance. Eur J Orthop Surg Traumatol. 2014;24(Suppl 1):S255–9.

Savage P, Sharkey R, Kua T, Schofield L, Richardson D, Panchmatia N, Papanastasopoulos P, Williams M, Falconer A, Power D, Arnold F, Ulbricht C. Malignant spinal cord compression: NICE guidance, improvements and challenges. QJM. 2014;107(4):277–82.

Sun JC, Xu T, Chen KF, Qian W, Liu K, Shi JG, Yuan W, Jia LS. Assessment of cauda equina syndrome progression pattern to improve diagnosis. Spine (Phila Pa 1976). 2014;39(7):596–602.

S. S. Goonewardene et al., *Basic Urological Management*,
https://doi.org/10.1007/978-3-319-98720-0_25

26 Urethral Strictures

Definition

- Narrowing of the urethra.
- The urethra is composed of bulbo-urethra, prostate and membranous urethra.
- Impairs urinary flow resulting in LUTS, spraying or spltting of the stream.
- Patient will often describe having to strain passing urine, and slow emptying, with a residual volume.
- Patients may also present in retention of urine.

Causes

- Infection - UTTS, STIs.
- Urethritis - non infectious.
- BXO.
- Trauma - blunt or penetrating.
- Post cystoscopy/instrumentation.
- Pelvic fracture disrupting the urethra.
- Post hypospadias repair.
- (Latini et al)

History

- History: IPSS score, LUTS (Storage and voiding symptoms), back pain.
- Spraying.
- Urinary frequency, urgency.
- Dysuria.
- Recurrent urinary tract infection.
- Inability to completely empty the bladder.
- Retention, weak stream, straining.
- (Mundi et al, Oelke et al)

S. S. Goonewardene et al., *Basic Urological Management*,
https://doi.org/10.1007/978-3-319-98720-0_26

Examination

- Abdomen: palpable masses in flanks (renal mass/ hydronephrosis), flank tenderness (?stones), SPC mass (bladder-retention or tumour).
- Scrotal examination, review of external urethral meatus, ?stenosis, check for phimosis, assess and make sure it is not a penile cancer causing obstruction (mass in body or glans).
- DRE: size of prostate, consistency.

Investigations

- Identify it prior to retention.
- Urine analysis/culture.
- Uroflowmetry.
- Post void residual.
- Renal function,if abnormal USS KUB (look for hydronephrosis).
- Flexible cystoscopy-review position of stricture).
- Urethrogram.
- Oelke et al.

Outcome

- Decompress bladder if in retention-catheterise for at least 3 days post procedure, then weekly ISC. Use S dilatiors or an SPC if no haematuria.
- Await the urethrogram to delineate length and anatomy of the stricture.
- Short strictures-us S-dilators, hegarty dilators, or cluton sounds to open up urethra or optical urethrotome.
- Long strictures should be referred to the appropriate centre for urethroplasty.
- AUA Guidelines on male urethral strictures.

Suggested Reading

Latini JM, McAninch JW, Brandes SB, Chung JY, Rosenstein D. SIU/ICUD consultation on urethral strictures: epidemiology, etiology, anatomy, and nomenclature of urethral stenoses, strictures, and pelvic fracture urethral disruption injuries. Urology. 2014;83(3 Suppl):S1–7.

Mundy AR, Andrich DE. Urethral strictures. BJU Int. 2011;107(1):6–26.

Oelke M, Bachmann A, Descazeaud A, Emberton M, Gravas S, Michel MC, N'dow J, Nordling J, de la Rosette JJ. EAU guidelines on the treatment and follow-up of non-neurogenic male lower urinary tract symptoms including benign prostatic obstruction. Eur Urol. 2013;64(1):118–40.

27 Diagnostic Pathway for Urethral Strictures

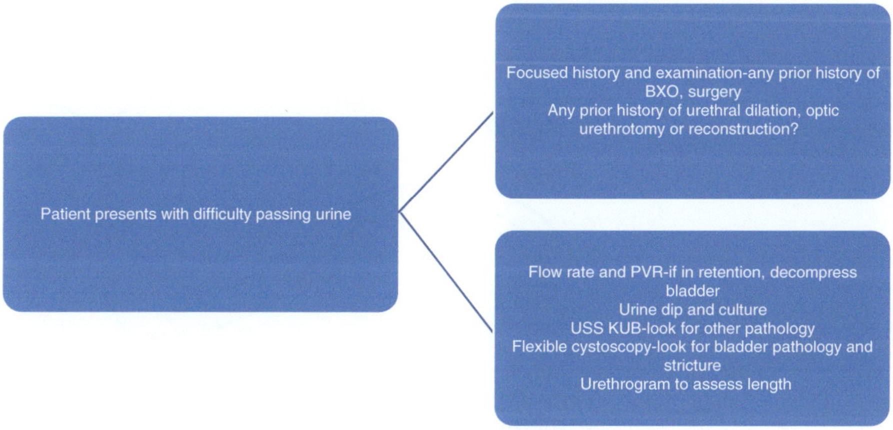

S. S. Goonewardene et al., *Basic Urological Management*,
https://doi.org/10.1007/978-3-319-98720-0_27

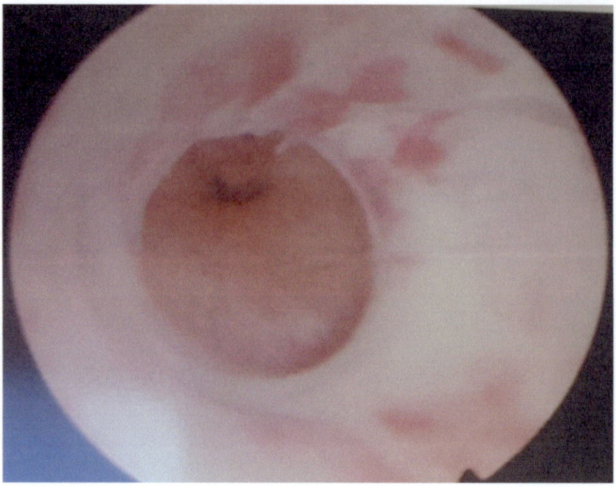

Fig. 27.1 Demonstrating a urethral stricture in a male—you can see the prostate behind the stricture

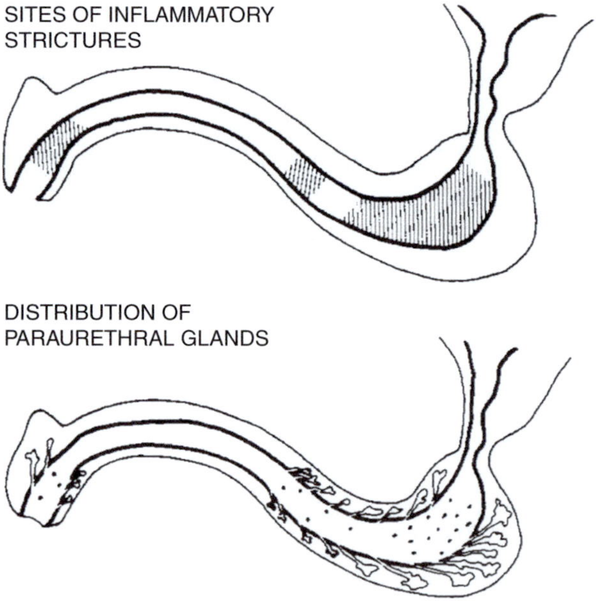

Fig. 27.2 Figure demonstrating sites of urethral stricture

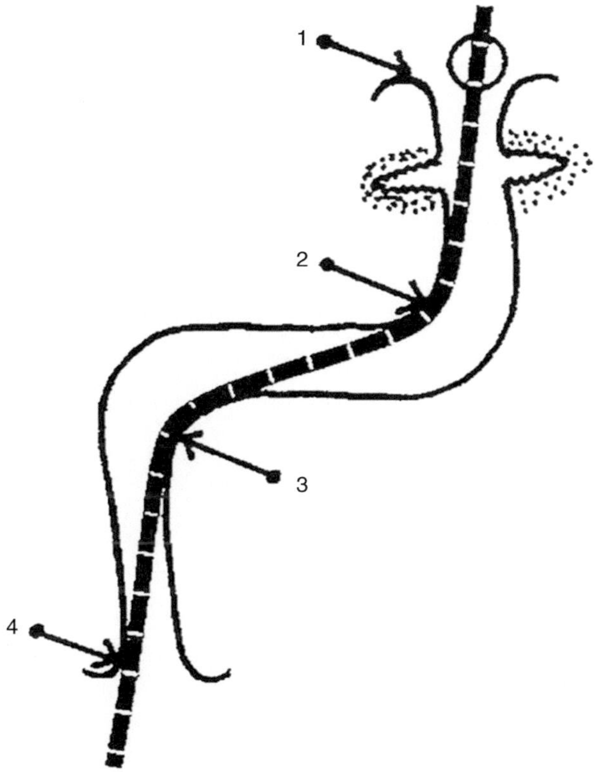

Fig. 27.3 Demonstrating sites of iatrogenic injury

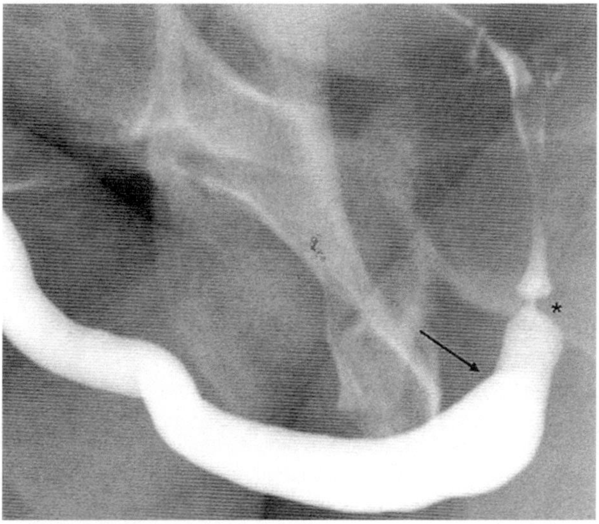

Fig. 27.4 Urethrogram demonstrating a urethral stricture

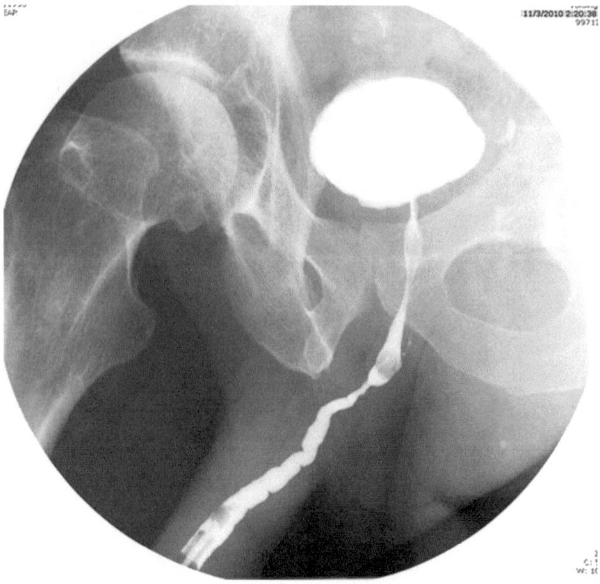

Fig. 27.5 Voiding Cystogram demonstrating urethral strictures

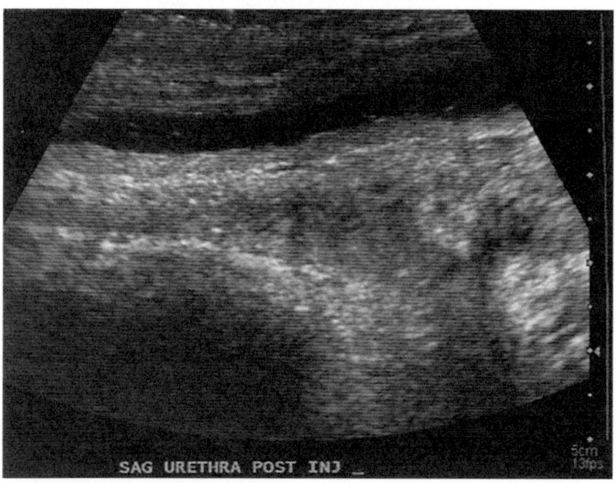

Fig. 27.6 Urethral stricture on US

Suggested Reading

Latini JM, McAninch JW, Brandes SB, Chung JY, Rosenstein D. SIU/ICUD consultation on urethral strictures: epidemiology, etiology, anatomy, and nomenclature of urethral stenoses, strictures, and pelvic fracture urethral disruption injuries. Urology. 2014;83(3 Suppl):S1–7.

Mundy AR, Andrich DE. Urethral strictures. BJU Int. 2011;107(1):6–26.

Oelke M, Bachmann A, Descazeaud A, Emberton M, Gravas S, Michel MC, N'dow J, Nordling J, de la Rosette JJ. EAU guidelines on the treatment and follow-up of non-neurogenic male lower urinary tract symptoms including benign prostatic obstruction. Eur Urol. 2013;64(1):118–40.

Management of Urethral Strictures

28

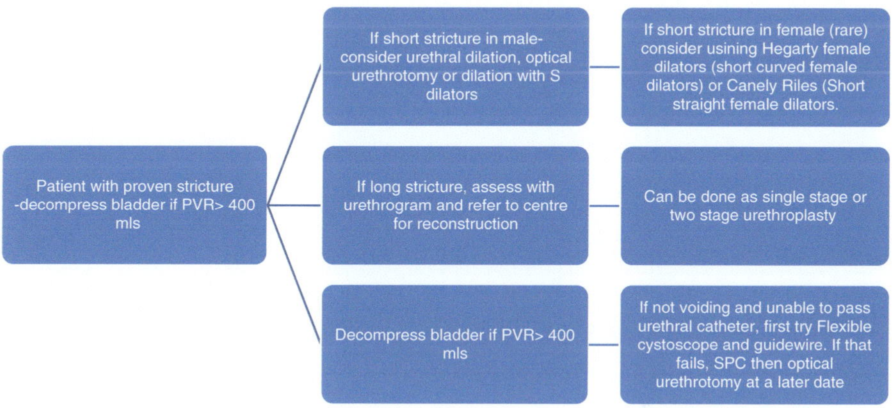

Suggested Reading

Latini JM, McAninch JW, Brandes SB, Chung JY, Rosenstein D. SIU/ICUD consultation on urethral strictures: epidemiology, etiology, anatomy, and nomenclature of urethral stenoses, strictures, and pelvic fracture urethral disruption injuries. Urology. 2014;83(3 Suppl):S1–7.

Mundy AR, Andrich DE. Urethral strictures. BJU Int. 2011;107(1):6–26.

Oelke M, Bachmann A, Descazeaud A, Emberton M, Gravas S, Michel MC, N'dow J, Nordling J, de la Rosette JJ. EAU guidelines on the treatment and follow-up of non-neurogenic male lower urinary tract symptoms including benign prostatic obstruction. Eur Urol. 2013;64(1):118–40.

S. S. Goonewardene et al., *Basic Urological Management*,
https://doi.org/10.1007/978-3-319-98720-0_28

29 Nocturnal Polyuria

Definition

- Passing large volumes of urine at night.
- Greater than 1/3rd of 24 hours output. (Madersbacher et al)
- Bladder diary (input, output, urgency, volume voided) required for diagnosis-mandatory.

Causes

- Diuretic medication.
- Caffeine related substances.
- Alcohol (diuretic).
- Excessive fluids before bedtime.
- Small bladder.
- Fluid redistribution from medical co-morbidities-DM, DI, Hypertension, CCF.

History

- History: IPSS score (storage and voiding sympts), LUTS. Back pain.
- Fluid intake and caffeine consumption.
- Medical co-morbidities: diabetes, SIADH.
- Nocturia and bladder diary with volume voided and at what time.

S. S. Goonewardene et al., *Basic Urological Management*,
https://doi.org/10.1007/978-3-319-98720-0_29

Examination

- Abdomen: palpable masses in flanks (renal mass/ hydronephrosis), flank tenderness (stones), SPC mass (bladder).
- Scrotal examination, review of external urethral meatus.
- DRE: prostate size and consistency.

Investigations

- Urine analysis-to review for infection (nitrites) and blood.
- Urine culture.
- Bladder diary, input, output and urgency.
- Uroflowmetry - check the maximum and average flow rate, voided volume.
- Post void residual.

Outcome

- Behavioural modification-restrict fluid intake, no fluids after 6 pm, cut out caffeine.
- Review the bladder diary in detail. Look at the number of voids, the frequency, how much are they passing, small volumes or larger volumes?
- Medical therapy-
  - First line anticholinergic therapy.
  - Second line: a dieuretic earier in the day.-to reduce nocturnal polyuria.
  - Third line: desmopressin (Drops the sodium-check sodium levels first).

Suggested Reading

Madersbacher S, Cornu JN. Nocturnal polyuria: it's all about definition, and be Patient! Eur Urol. 2013;63(3):548–50.

Oelke M, Bachmann A, Descazeaud A, Emberton M, Gravas S, Michel MC, N'dow J, Nordling J, de la Rosette JJ. EAU guidelines on the treatment and follow-up of non-neurogenic male lower urinary tract symptoms including benign prostatic obstruction. Eur Urol. 2013;64(1):118–40.

van Kerrebroeck P, Abrams P, Chaikin D, Donovan J, Fonda D, Jackson S, Jennum P, Johnson T, Lose G, Mattiasson A, Robertson G, Weiss J. The standardisation of terminology in nocturia: Report from the standardisation sub-committee of the International Continence Society. Neurourol Urodyn. 2002;21(2):179–83.

Diagnostic Pathway for Nocturnal Polyuria

30

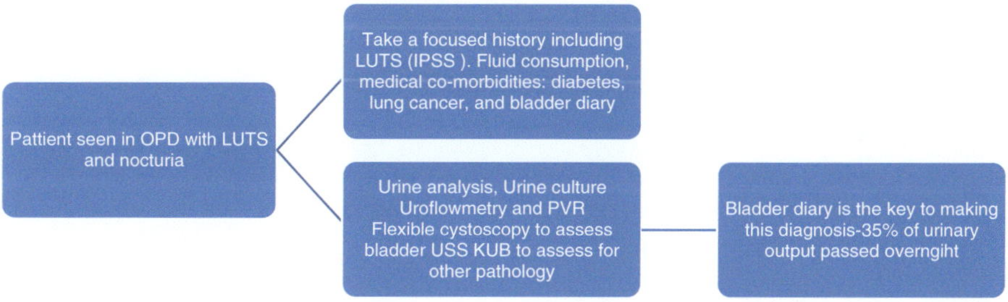

Suggested Reading

Madersbacher S, Cornu JN. Nocturnal polyuria: it's all about definition, and be Patient! Eur Urol. 2013;63(3):548–50.

Oelke M, Bachmann A, Descazeaud A, Emberton M, Gravas S, Michel MC, N'dow J, Nordling J, de la Rosette JJ. EAU guidelines on the treatment and follow-up of non-neurogenic male lower urinary tract symptoms including benign prostatic obstruction. Eur Urol. 2013;64(1):118–40.

van Kerrebroeck P, Abrams P, Chaikin D, Donovan J, Fonda D, Jackson S, Jennum P, Johnson T, Lose G, Mattiasson A, Robertson G, Weiss J. The standardisation of terminology in nocturia: Report from the standardisation sub-committee of the International Continence Society. Neurourol Urodyn. 2002;21(2):179–83.

S. S. Goonewardene et al., *Basic Urological Management*,
https://doi.org/10.1007/978-3-319-98720-0_30

31 Management Pathway for Nocturnal Polyuria

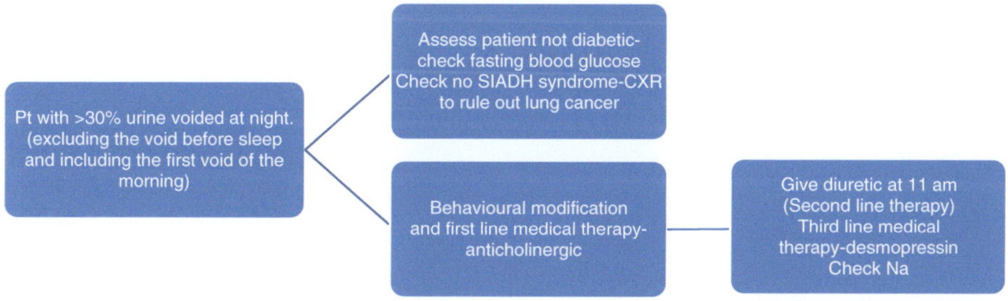

Suggested Reading

Madersbacher S, Cornu JN. Nocturnal polyuria: it's all about definition, and be Patient! Eur Urol. 2013;63(3):548–50.

Oelke M, Bachmann A, Descazeaud A, Emberton M, Gravas S, Michel MC, N'dow J, Nordling J, de la Rosette JJ. EAU guidelines on the treatment and follow-up of non-neurogenic male lower urinary tract symptoms including benign prostatic obstruction. Eur Urol. 2013;64(1):118–40.

van Kerrebroeck P, Abrams P, Chaikin D, Donovan J, Fonda D, Jackson S, Jennum P, Johnson T, Lose G, Mattiasson A, Robertson G, Weiss J. The standardisation of terminology in nocturia: Report from the standardisation sub-committee of the International Continence Society. Neurourol Urodyn. 2002;21(2):179–83.

S. S. Goonewardene et al., *Basic Urological Management*,
https://doi.org/10.1007/978-3-319-98720-0_31

Dysuria

32

Definition

- Pain/burning during urination.
- May also be associated with other symptoms e.g. LUTS.
- Often the result of urinary stasis and infection as a result of that.
- Bacturia is the presence of bacteria in the urinary.
- With the UTI, there are 10^5 colony forming units on a culture plate (Johansen et al).
- Look for an anatomical, obstructive or infectious cause.

Causes

- Urinary tract obstruction: Bladder outflow obstruction-BPH, prostate cancer, urethral stricture, obstructing stone.
- Infections: UTI, cystitis, prostatitis, urethritis, pyelonephritis, STIS.
- Stones: Renal stones, ureteric or bladder, prostatic calculi.
- Schistosoma, trichomonas.
- Neoplasia: Bladder cancer, prostatic cancer, urethral cancer.
- Vesico-ureteric reflux.
- (Michels et al)

History

- History: IPSS score, LUTS.
- Urinary frequency, urgency.
- Dysuria-extent and duration, STIs.
- Recurrent urinary tract infections.
- Inability to completely empty the bladder.
- Retention, sepsis, fevers, rigors, abdominal pain.
- Prior treatment-antibiotics, imaging.
- (Naber et al)

S. S. Goonewardene et al., *Basic Urological Management*,
https://doi.org/10.1007/978-3-319-98720-0_32

Examination

- Abdomen: flank tenderness (stones), palpable bladder (retention), ?bladder mass.
- Scrotal examination, review of external urethral meatus.
- DRE: anal tone, sensation.

Investigations

- Urine analysis/culture-check past cultures.
- Uroflowmetry.
- Post void residual.
- USS KUB/ CT KUB if stones suspected-look for stones obstructing the urinary system needing either stent or nephrostomy.
- Unobstructing stones can also cause infections and dysuria.
- Renal function.
- Flexible cystoscopy-to rule out bladder tumour, bladder stones.
- (Naber et al)

Outcome

- If recurrent UTIS-consider lifestyle measures, and a low dose of prophylactic antibiotic.
- If stones-make sure patient is not obstructed and follow stones pathway-defntitive treatment for stone may be ESWL, ureteroscopy or PCNL.
- If LUTS from BPH, medical therapy as 1st line, then surgical management.
- If bladder tumour, book for TURBT if fit for surgery-bladder tumour pathway.
- IF Prostate cancer-follow prostate cancer pathway.

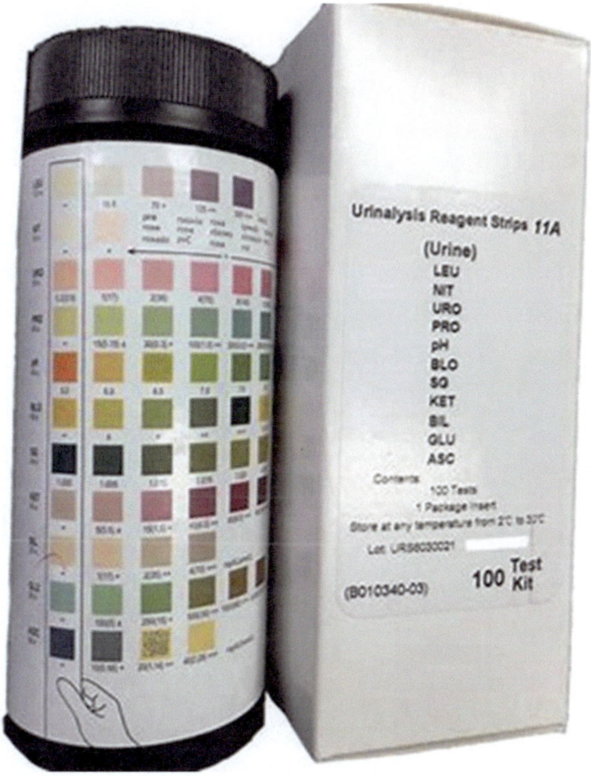

Fig. 32.1 Urine dip sticks

Suggested Reading

Johansen TE, Botto H, Cek M, Grabe M, Tenke P, Wagenlehner FM, Naber KG. Critical review of current definitions of urinary tract infections and proposal of an EAU/ESIU classification system. Int J Antimicrob Agents. 2011;38(Suppl):64–70.

Michels TC, Sands JE. Dysuria: evaluation and differential diagnosis in adults. Am Fam Physician. 2015;92(9):778–86.

Naber KG, Bergman B, Bishop MC, Bjerklund-Johansen TE, Botto H, Lobel B, Jinenez Cruz F, Selvaggi FP, Urinary Tract Infection (UTI) Working Group of the Health Care Office (HCO) of the European Association of Urology (EAU). EAU guidelines for the management of urinary and male genital tract infections. Urinary Tract Infection (UTI) Working Group of the Health Care Office (HCO) of the European Association of Urology (EAU). Eur Urol. 2001;40(5):576–88.

Diagnostic Pathway for Dysuria

33

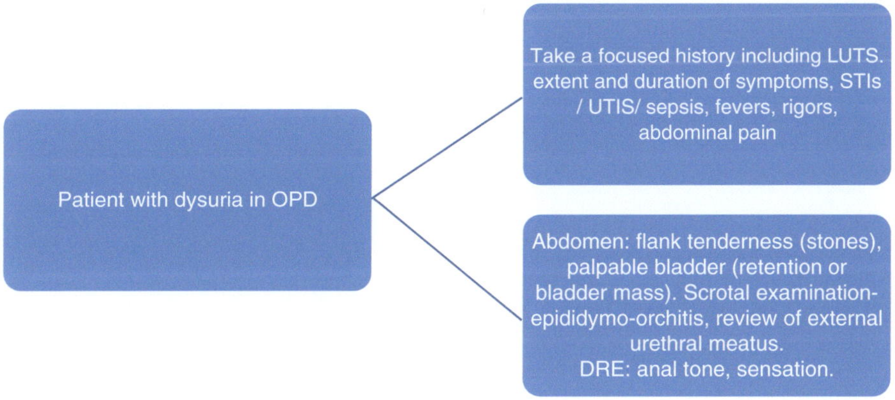

Suggested Reading

Johansen TE, Botto H, Cek M, Grabe M, Tenke P, Wagenlehner FM, Naber KG. Critical review of current definitions of urinary tract infections and proposal of an EAU/ESIU classification system. Int J Antimicrob Agents. 2011;38(Suppl):64–70.

Michels TC, Sands JE. Dysuria: Evaluation and Differential Diagnosis in Adults. Am Fam Physician. 2015;92(9):778–86.

Naber KG, Bergman B, Bishop MC, Bjerklund-Johansen TE, Botto H, Lobel B, Jinenez Cruz F, Selvaggi FP, Urinary Tract Infection (UTI) Working Group of the Health Care Office (HCO) of the European Association of Urology (EAU). EAU guidelines for the management of urinary and male genital tract infections. Urinary Tract Infection (UTI) Working Group of the Health Care Office (HCO) of the European Association of Urology (EAU). Eur Urol. 2001;40(5):576–88.

S. S. Goonewardene et al., *Basic Urological Management*,
https://doi.org/10.1007/978-3-319-98720-0_33

Management Pathways for Dysuria: Recurrent UTIS

34

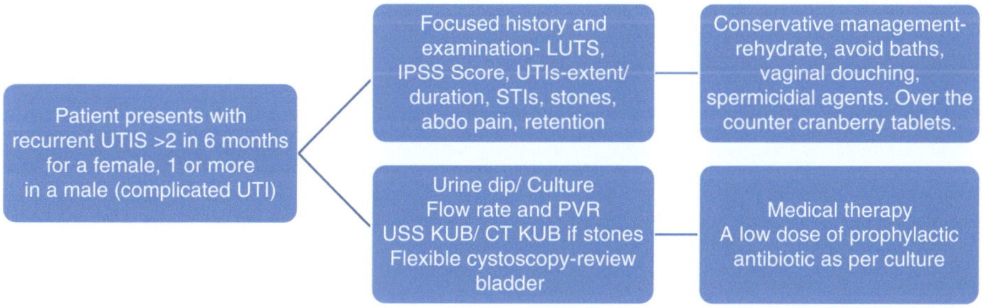

Suggested Reading

Michels TC, Sands JE. Dysuria: evaluation and differential diagnosis in adults. Am Fam Physician. 2015;92(9):778–86.

Naber KG, Bergman B, Bishop MC, Bjerklund-Johansen TE, Botto H, Lobel B, Jinenez Cruz F, Selvaggi FP. Urinary Tract Infection (UTI) Working Group of the Health Care Office (HCO) of the European Association of Urology (EAU). EAU guidelines for the management of urinary and male genital tract infections. Urinary Tract Infection (UTI) Working Group of the Health Care Office (HCO) of the European Association of Urology (EAU). Eur Urol. 2001;40(5):576–88.

Johansen TE, Botto H, Cek M, Grabe M, Tenke P, Wagenlehner FM, Naber KG. Critical review of current definitions of urinary tract infections and proposal of an EAU/ESIU classification system. Int J Antimicrob Agents. 2011;38:64–70.

S. S. Goonewardene et al., *Basic Urological Management*,
https://doi.org/10.1007/978-3-319-98720-0_34

Sepsis

35

Definition

- Sepsis-the bodys' reaction to infection.
- The underlying pathology is one of organ hypoperfusion, hypotension and increased vascular permeability.
- Severe sepsis-sepsis strong enough to cause SIRS.
- Septic shock-shock caused by hypoperfusion of organs.
- (Singler et al)

Causes

- Urological sources of sepsis
- Urinary tract infections, pyelonephritis, cystitis.
- Stones/ Obstructive stones-usually with associated hydronephrosis.
- Perinephris abcess, pyonephrosis, renal abcess, pelvic abcess/ collection.
- Ureteral obstruction-tumour, stones, external compression.
- Bladder outflow obstruction, retention.
- Mutiple attempts at catheterisation.
- Moore et al.

S. S. Goonewardene et al., *Basic Urological Management*,
https://doi.org/10.1007/978-3-319-98720-0_35

History

- Sepsis-duration, fevers, rigors.
- LUTS: Urinary frequency, urgency, nocturia, terminal dribbling, strain, weak stream, incomplete emptying.
- Pain-abdominal.
- Dysuria-extent and duration.
- Recurrent urinary tract infection, stones, BOO.
- Inability to completely empty the bladder.
- Prior treatment-antibiotcs, imaging.
- LTC-last change.

Examination

- Look for the cause of sepsis.
- Assess via an ABCDE approach.
- Note Capilllary refill time and observations.
- Assess chest for repiratory causes.
- Assess abdomen-? obstructing stones,? retention,? post op, GI cause of sepsis.

Investigations

- IV access x2, widebore.
- Get antibiotics in early and start fluid resuscitation.
- Bloods including FBC, U+Es, CRP, LFTs, clotting, G+S.
- Blood cultures, urine culture.
- ABG for lactate.
- CT scan.

Outcome

- Get patient to ITU/HDU.
- Management definitive problem causing sepsis.
- If obstructing stone, nephrostomy.
- If in retention, catheterise.
- Strict fluid balence.
- Daily microbiology review.
- (Cawcutt et al)

Suggested Reading

Cawcutt KA, Peters SG. Severe sepsis and septic shock: clinical overview and update on management. Mayo Clin Proc. 2014;89(11):1572–8.

Moore LJ, Moore FA. Early diagnosis and evidence-based care of surgical sepsis. J Intensive Care Med. 2013;28(2):107–17.

Singer M, Deutschman CS, Seymour CW, Shankar-Hari M, Annane D, Bauer M, Bellomo R, Bernard GR, Chiche JD, Coopersmith CM, Hotchkiss RS, Levy MM, Marshall JC, Martin GS, Opal SM, Rubenfeld GD, van der Poll T, Vincent JL, Angus DC. The Third International Consensus Definitions for Sepsis and Septic Shock (Sepsis-3). JAMA. 2016;315(8):801–10.

Diagnostic and Management Pathway for Sepsis

36

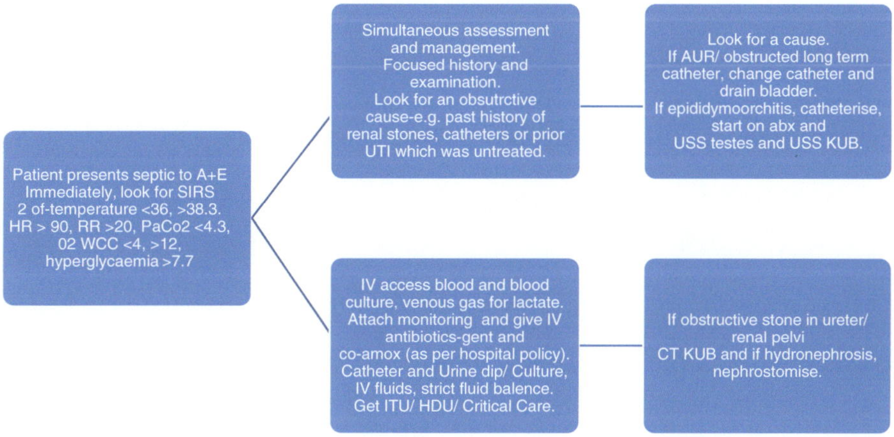

Suggested Reading

Cawcutt KA, Peters SG. Severe sepsis and septic shock: clinical overview and update on management. Mayo Clin Proc. 2014;89(11):1572–8.

Moore LJ, Moore FA. Early diagnosis and evidence-based care of surgical sepsis. J Intensive Care Med. 2013;28(2):107–17.

Singer M, Deutschman CS, Seymour CW, Shankar-Hari M, Annane D, Bauer M, Bellomo R, Bernard GR, Chiche JD, Coopersmith CM, Hotchkiss RS, Levy MM, Marshall JC, Martin GS, Opal SM, Rubenfeld GD, van der Poll T, Vincent JL, Angus DC. The third international consensus definitions for sepsis and septic shock (Sepsis-3). JAMA. 2016;315(8):801–10.

S. S. Goonewardene et al., *Basic Urological Management*,
https://doi.org/10.1007/978-3-319-98720-0_36

Acute Pyelonephritis

37

Definition

- Infection of the renal pelvis and renal parenchyma.
- Look for an underlying urological cause.
- Is the patient obstructed?
- Are there stones?
- Are they in retention?
- Do they have a long term catheter?
- Is there a TCC in the ureter?

Causes

- Common causes: E.coli, Proteus, KLebisiella, Enterococcus. (Prabhu et al)
- Risk factors: structurally abnormal urinary tract, obstruction, (BPH, prostate cancer), renal stones, instrumentation, forerign bodies e.g. stents, pregnancy, diabetes, immunosupresion, neuropathic bladder.
- Ascending: bLadder outflow obstruction-BPH, + prostate cancer, urethral stricture.
- Descending: stones, PUJO (obstruction).
- UTI, Cystitis, prostatitis, urethritis, pyelonephritis, STI, renal stones, ureteric or bladder stones.

S. S. Goonewardene et al., *Basic Urological Management*,
https://doi.org/10.1007/978-3-319-98720-0_37

History

- History: IPSS score, LUTS.
- Irritative symptoms, urinary frequency, urgency.
- Dysuria-extent and duration.
- Recurrent urinary tract infection.
- Inability to completely empty the bladder.
- Retention.
- Prior treatment-antibiotcs, imaging
- (Naber et al, EAU Guidelines), Lane et al.

Examination

- Abdomen: flank tenderness (stones), palpable bladder (retention), ? bladder mass.
- Scrotal examination, review of external urethral meatus.
- DRE: anal tone, sensation.

Investigations

- Urine analysis/ culture.
- Uroflowmetry-is the bladder draining.
- Post void residual-do they have a stricture preventing bladder drainage.
- USS KUB/ CT KUB if stones suspected.
- Renal function-do they have an obstructive uropathy.
- Flexible cystoscopy-bladder stones or an tumour-do if blood on dip.
- (EAU Guidelines)

Outcome

- Decompress bladder if in retention-catheterise for at least 3 days.
- If stones and obstructed-decompress system with nephrostomy or stent, then definitive stone management later-PCNL or URS.
- If LUTS and in retention and > 1L drained, for TURP.
- If bladder stone-put patient on abx and catheterise, stone punch to extract.
- Identify and treat diabetes.

Suggested Reading

Lane DR, Takhar SS. Diagnosis and management of urinary tract infection and pyelonephritis. Emerg Med Clin North Am. 2011;29(3):539–52.

Naber KG, Bergman B, Bishop MC, Bjerklund-Johansen TE, Botto H, Lobel B, Jinenez Cruz F, Selvaggi FP, EAU guidelines for the management of urinary and male genital tract infections. Urinary Tract Infection (UTI) Working Group of the Health Care Office (HCO) of the European Association of Urology (EAU). Eur Urol. 2001;40(5):576–88.

Prabhu A, Taylor P, Konecny P, Brown MA. Pyelonephritis: what are the present day causative organisms and antibiotic susceptibilities? Nephrology (Carlton). 2013;18(6):463–7.

Chronic Pyelonephritis

38

Definition

- Long standing (> 3 months) Infection of the renal pelvis and renal parenchyma causing inflammation and fibrosis.
- Continuing pyogenic infection of the kidney.
- It can cause renal scarring (upper pole typically) which may result in CKD and ESRF requiring transplant.

Causes

- Common causes: E.coli, Proteus, Klebisiella, Enterococcus.
- Risk factors: structurally abnormal urinary tract, VUR, obstruction, (BPH< prostate cancer), renal stones, instrumentation, foreign bodies e.g. stents, pregnancy, diabetes, immunosupresion, neuropathic bladder.
- Ascending: bladder outflow obstruction-BPH, prostate cancer, urethral stricture.
- Descending: stones, PUJO (obstruction).
- Infective causses: UTI, cystitis, prostatitis, urethritis, pyelonephritis, STI, renal stones, ureteric or bladder stones.

S. S. Goonewardene et al., *Basic Urological Management*,
https://doi.org/10.1007/978-3-319-98720-0_38

History

- History: Sexual activity. Pregnancy if female.
- Patient may have no symptoms.
- Backache
- Storage and voiding LUTS, fatigue, decreased libido, dysuria.
- Abdominal pain/ flank pain, fever.
- Recurrent urinary tract infection.
- Prior treatment-antibiotcs, imaging.
- Childhood history of VUR, ureteric re-implantation.

Examination

- Abdomen: flank tenderness (stones), palpable bladder (retention), ? bladder mass.
- Scrotal examination, review of external urethral meatus.
- DRE: anal tone, sensation.

Investigations

- Obs-is there high blood pressure? -intrinsic renal disease.
- Urine analysis/ culture-is pyuria present?-an indication of infection.
- Uroflowmetry.
- Video urodynamics for neuropathic bladder
- Post void residual -are they emptying
- USS KUB/ CT KUB if stones suspected or pyonphrosis
- Renal function (CKD), HB (anaemia)
- MAG 3 renogram to review split renal function/ DMSA for static renal function

Outcome

- Approriate antibiotic therapy as per culture, in most hospitals, give gentamicin.
- IV access, fluids
- Catheter to drain bladder and monitor urine output.
- Treat the cause-if obstructed, drain bladder, if stones, treat stones.
- CKD-admit an get nephrology review.
- Control diabetes.

Suggested Reading

Blanc AL, Vialle B, Lemaire X, Poissy J, Melliez H, François P, Senneville E, Yazdanpanah Y. Chronic pyelonephritis and xanthogranulomatous pyelonephritis. Urol J. 2007;4(3):169–73.

Naber KG, Bergman B, Bishop MC, Bjerklund-Johansen TE, Botto H, Lobel B, Jinenez Cruz F, Selvaggi FP, EAU guidelines for the management of urinary and male genital tract infections. Urinary Tract Infection (UTI) Working Group of the Health Care Office (HCO) of the European Association of Urology (EAU). Eur Urol. 2001;40(5):576–88.

Diagnostic Pathway for Pyelonephritis

39

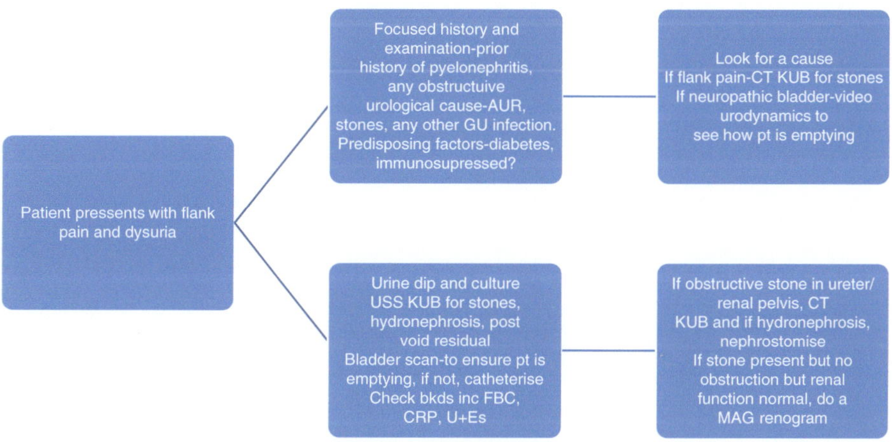

Fig. 39.1 CT demonstrating severe acute bacterial pyelonephritis

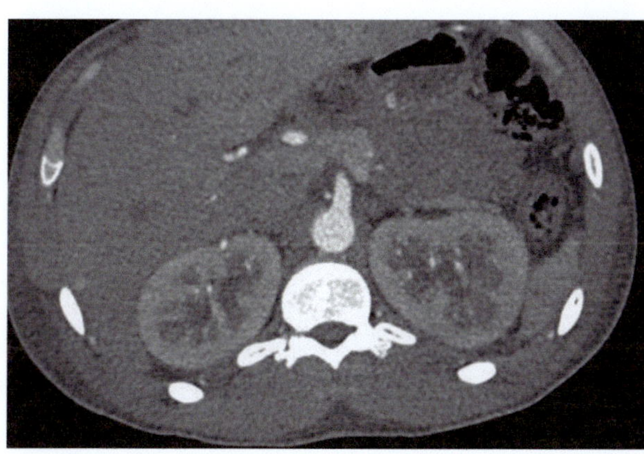

S. S. Goonewardene et al., *Basic Urological Management*,
https://doi.org/10.1007/978-3-319-98720-0_39

Suggested Reading

Blanc AL, Vialle B, Lemaire X, Poissy J, Melliez H, François P, Senneville E, Yazdanpanah Y. Chronic pyelonephritis and xanthogranulomatous pyelonephritis. Urol J. 2007;4(3):169–73.

Naber KG, Bergman B, Bishop MC, Bjerklund-Johansen TE, Botto H, Lobel B, Jinenez Cruz F, Selvaggi FP, EAU guidelines for the management of urinary and male genital tract infections. Urinary Tract Infection (UTI) Working Group of the Health Care Office (HCO) of the European Association of Urology (EAU). Eur Urol. 2001;40(5):576–88.

40 Management Pathway for Pyelonephritis

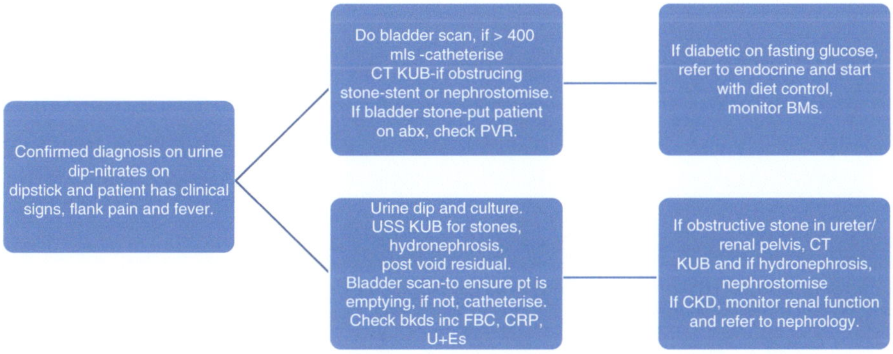

Suggested Reading

Blanc AL, Vialle B, Lemaire X, Poissy J, Melliez H, François P, Senneville E, Yazdanpanah Y. Chronic pyelonephritis and xanthogranulomatous pyelonephritis. Urol J. 2007;4(3):169–73.

Naber KG, Bergman B, Bishop MC, Bjerklund-Johansen TE, Botto H, Lobel B, Jinenez Cruz F, Selvaggi FP, EAU guidelines for the management of urinary and male genital tract infections. Urinary Tract Infection (UTI) Working Group of the Health Care Office (HCO) of the European Association of Urology (EAU). Eur Urol. 2001;40(5):576–88.

S. S. Goonewardene et al., *Basic Urological Management*, https://doi.org/10.1007/978-3-319-98720-0_40

41 Cystitis

Definition

- Infection and inflammation of the urinary bladder.
- Uncomplicated-in the presence of a structurally normal urinary tract
- Complicated-presence of infection in the male urinary system, or in a anatomically abnormal urinary tract
- Patients often present with recurrent episodes, requiring treatment.

Causes

- (Colgan et al)
- Intercourse
- Short urethra
- Recurrent UTIS
- Bladder stones
- Diabetes
- BOO
- Diaphragm contraceptive
- Poor hygiene
- Presence of foreskin
- LTC

S. S. Goonewardene et al., *Basic Urological Management*,
https://doi.org/10.1007/978-3-319-98720-0_41

History

- History: sexual history, LUTS.
- Abdominal / SPC pain.
- Urinary frequency, urgency, haematuria (look for malignancy).
- Dysuria-extent and duration.
- Recurrent urinary tract infection.
- Inability to completely empty the bladder-LTC
- Retention, stones.
- Prior treatment-antibiotcs, imaging, surgery.

Examination

- Abdomen: flank tenderness (stones) or masses, palpable bladder (retention), ? bladder mass.
- Tenderness in supra-pubic region-cystitis?
- Scrotal examination, review of external urethral meatus.
- Cathter size gauge, colour of urine, blockages, last changed. Position-urethral or SPC.
- DRE: size and consistency of prostate, volume.

Investigations

- Urine analysis/ culture.
- Uroflowmetry-check bladder is emptying.
- Post void residual-check < 200 mls.
- USS KUB/ CT KUB if stones suspected.
- Renal function.
- Flexible cystoscopy-look for hunners ulcers and glomerulations, signs of interstitial cystitis, look to exclude malignancy.

Outcome

- Treat infections according to sensitivity results.
- Put patient on empirical antibiotics until cultures come through.
- Correct surgical/ anatomical causes e.g. surgery for VUR, BOO.
- Encourage oral intake of water.
- OTC cranberry tablets or hiprex.
- Make sure patient has good hygeiene measures.
- Ensure LTCs are in the correct position and draining properly.

Suggested Reading

Colgan R, Williams M. Diagnosis and treatment of acute uncomplicated cystitis. Am Fam Physician. 2011;84(7):771–6.

Gupta K, Hooton TM, Naber KG, Wullt B, Colgan R, Miller LG, Moran GJ, Nicolle LE, Raz R, Schaeffer AJ, Soper DE. International clinical practice guidelines for the treatment of acute uncomplicated cystitis and pyelonephritis in women: a 2010 update by the Infectious Diseases Society of America and the European Society for Microbiology and Infectious Diseases. Clin Infect Dis. 2011;52(5):e103–20.

Yamamoto S, Higuchi Y, Nojima M. Current therapy of acute uncomplicated cystitis. Int J Urol. 2010;17(5):450–6.

Diagnostic Pathway for Cystitis

42

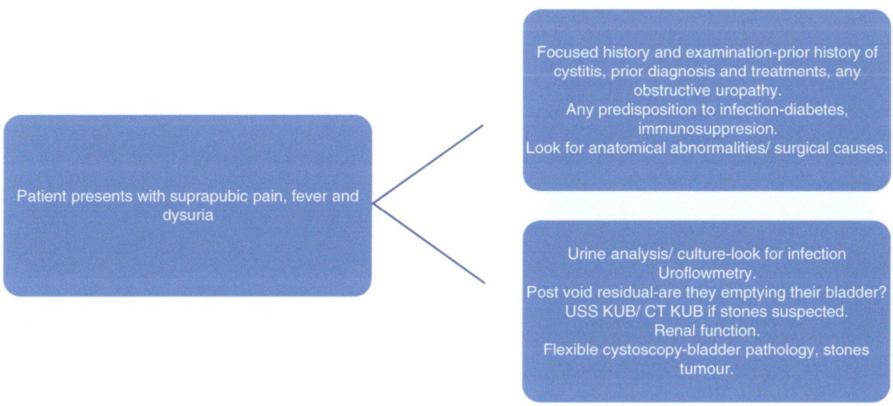

Suggested Reading

Colgan R, Williams M. Diagnosis and treatment of acute uncomplicated cystitis. Am Fam Physician. 2011;84(7):771–6.

Gupta K, Hooton TM, Naber KG, Wullt B, Colgan R, Miller LG, Moran GJ, Nicolle LE, Raz R, Schaeffer AJ, Soper DE. International clinical practice guidelines for the treatment of acute uncomplicated cystitis and pyelonephritis in women: a 2010 update by the Infectious Diseases Society of America and the European Society for Microbiology and Infectious Diseases. Clin Infect Dis. 2011;52(5):e103–20.

Yamamoto S, Higuchi Y, Nojima M. Current therapy of acute uncomplicated cystitis. Int J Urol. 2010;17(5):450–6.

S. S. Goonewardene et al., *Basic Urological Management*,
https://doi.org/10.1007/978-3-319-98720-0_42

Management Pathway for Cystitis

43

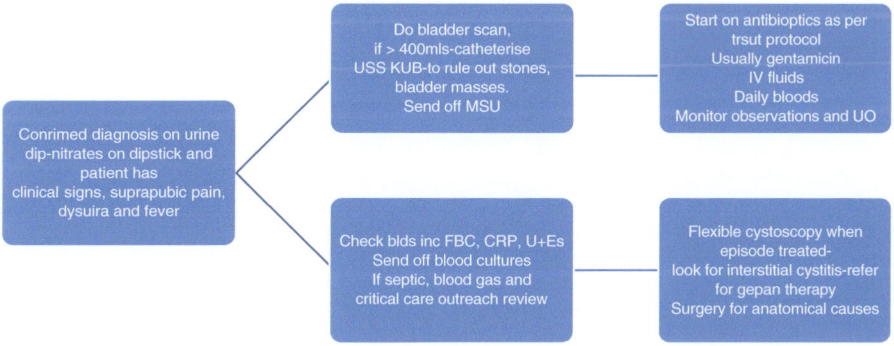

Suggested Reading

Colgan R, Williams M. Diagnosis and treatment of acute uncomplicated cystitis. Am Fam Physician. 2011;84(7):771–6.

Gupta K, Hooton TM, Naber KG, Wullt B, Colgan R, Miller LG, Moran GJ, Nicolle LE, Raz R, Schaeffer AJ, Soper DE. International clinical practice guidelines for the treatment of acute uncomplicated cystitis and pyelonephritis in women: a 2010 update by the Infectious Diseases Society of America and the European Society for Microbiology and Infectious Diseases. Clin Infect Dis. 2011;52(5):e103–20.

Yamamoto S, Higuchi Y, Nojima M. Current therapy of acute uncomplicated cystitis. Int J Urol. 2010;17(5):450–6.

S. S. Goonewardene et al., *Basic Urological Management*,
https://doi.org/10.1007/978-3-319-98720-0_43

44 Pyonephrosis

Definition

- A collection of white bloods cells, pus and bacteria in the collecting system.
- Main factors causing it: bacteria in the upper urinary tract and obstruction.
- Risk factors: immunosuppresion, diabetes, abnormal urinary tract anatomy (horseshoe kidneys, stones, transplant kidney, malignancy).
- Pyonephrosis requires immediate drainage with either ureteric stent or nephrostomy.

Causes

- Causes: ascending infections from bladder, E. Coli, Klesiella, Proteus, Candida.
- Colonisation of LTC.
- BOO.
- Post surgery, cystoscopy, ureteroscopy or PCNL.
- Hydronephrosis.
- Anatomically abnormal urinary tract, obstructive stone.
- (Sow et al)

S. S. Goonewardene et al., *Basic Urological Management*,
https://doi.org/10.1007/978-3-319-98720-0_44

History

- History: LUTS, urinary tract obstruction.
- Nausea and vomiting.
- Urinary frequency, urgency, incomplete emptying.
- Dysuria-extent and duration.
- Fever chills, flank pain.
- Prior treatment-antibiotcs, imaging.
- Immunosuppresion, diabetes.
- (EAU Guidelines)

Examination

- Review for sepsis.
- Abdomen: flank tenderness (stones), Palpable flanks/ back mass (abcess), palpable bladder (retention),? bladder mass.
- Scrotal examination, review of external urethral meatus.
- DRE: Size, consistency and volume of prostate, anal tone, sensation.

Investigations

- ABCDE approach
- IV line
- IV abx-Usually gentamicim if no renal impairment
- Fluid resuscitate
- Urine analysis/ culture
- Catheter and strict fluid balence
- Bloods in FBC U+Es and clotting CRP, ABG
- CT KUB

Outcome

- Nephrostomy or stent insertion under IV abx cover
- ITU/ HDU care
- MAG 3 renogram at a later date-kidney may become none functional and require nephrectomy later on

Suggested Reading

Ludvigson AE, Beaule LT. Urologic emergencies. Surg Clin North Am. 2016;96(3):407–24.

Naber KG, Bergman B, Bishop MC, Bjerklund-Johansen TE, Botto H, Lobel B, Jinenez Cruz F, Selvaggi FP. EAU guidelines for the management of urinary and male genital tract infections. Urinary Tract Infection (UTI) Working Group of the Health Care Office (HCO) of the European Association of Urology (EAU). Eur Urol. 2001;40(5):576–88.

Sow Y, Fall B, Sarr A, Thiam A, Diao B, Fall PA, Ndoye AK, Ba M, Diagne BA. Pyonephrosis: 44 cases in Senegal. Med Trop (Mars). 2011;71(5):495–8.

45 Diagnosis of Pyonephrosis

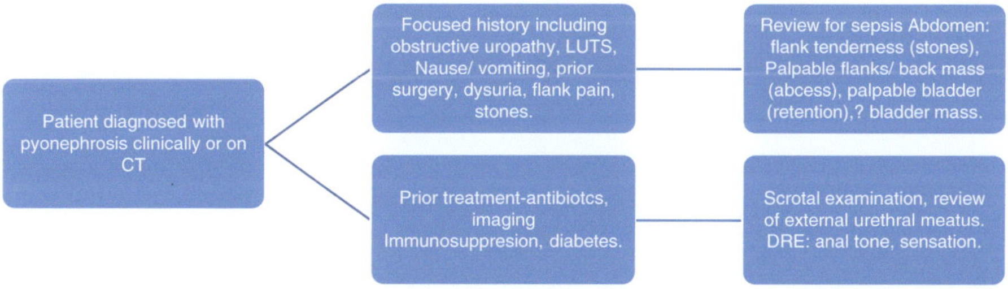

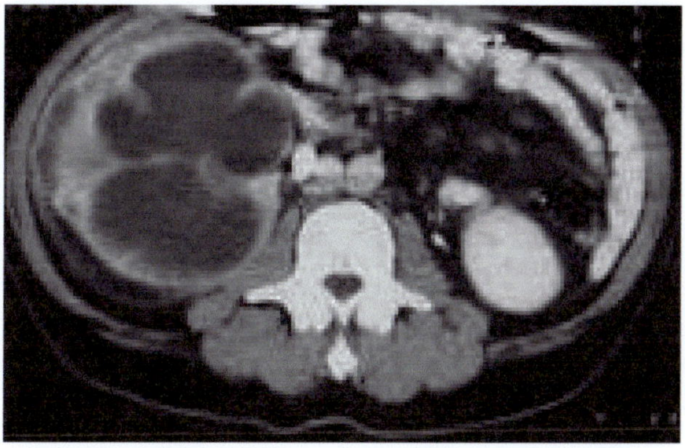

Fig. 45.1 CT demonstrating pyonephrosis

S. S. Goonewardene et al., *Basic Urological Management*,
https://doi.org/10.1007/978-3-319-98720-0_45

Suggested Reading

Ludvigson AE, Beaule LT. Urologic emergencies. Surg Clin North Am. 2016;96(3):407–24.

Naber KG, Bergman B, Bishop MC, Bjerklund-Johansen TE, Botto H, Lobel B, Jinenez Cruz F, Selvaggi FP. EAU guidelines for the management of urinary and male genital tract infections. Urinary Tract Infection (UTI) Working Group of the Health Care Office (HCO) of the European Association of Urology (EAU). Eur Urol. 2001;40(5):576–88.

Sow Y, Fall B, Sarr A, Thiam A, Diao B, Fall PA, Ndoye AK, Ba M, Diagne BA. Pyonephrosis: 44 cases in Senegal. Med Trop (Mars). 2011;71(5):495–8.

Management Pathway for Pyonephrosis 46

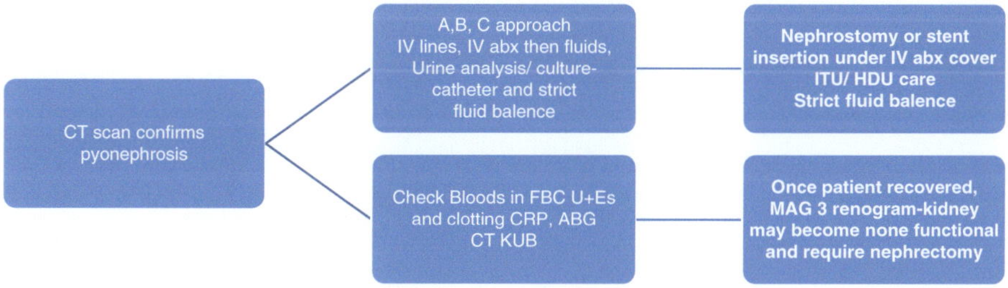

Suggested Reading

Ludvigson AE, Beaule LT. Urologic emergencies. Surg Clin North Am. 2016;96(3):407–24.

Naber KG, Bergman B, Bishop MC, Bjerklund-Johansen TE, Botto H, Lobel B, Jinenez Cruz F, Selvaggi FP. EAU guidelines for the management of urinary and male genital tract infections. Urinary Tract Infection (UTI) Working Group of the Health Care Office (HCO) of the European Association of Urology (EAU). Eur Urol. 2001;40(5):576–88.

Sow Y, Fall B, Sarr A, Thiam A, Diao B, Fall PA, Ndoye AK, Ba M, Diagne BA. Pyonephrosis: 44 cases in Senegal. Med Trop (Mars). 2011;71(5):495–8.

S. S. Goonewardene et al., *Basic Urological Management*,
https://doi.org/10.1007/978-3-319-98720-0_46

Perinephric Abcess

47

Definition

- A collection of pus in the perinephric space.
- It can rupture through the fascia to become a paranephric abcess.
- Patients often present as critically sick into A+E.
- This is a condition that must be managed quickly and efficiently
- (Meng et al)

Causes

- Common causes: E.coli, Proteus and Staph, Klebsiella, Proteus, Enterobacter, Pseudomonas, serratia.
- Urinary tract obstruction or spread from blood
- Perforation of urinary system-post instrumentation
- Risk factors: structurally abnormal urinary tract, obstruction, (BPH, prostate cancer), renal stones, instrumentation, foreign bodies e.g. stents, pregnancy, diabetes, immunosupresion, neuropathic bladder.
- Ascending: bladder outflow obstruction-BPH, prostate cancer, urethral stricture.
- Descending: stones, PUJO (obstruction).
- UTI, Cystitis, prostatitis, urethritis, pyelonephritis, STI, renal stones, ureteric or bladder stones.
- (Gardiner et al)

S. S. Goonewardene et al., *Basic Urological Management*,
https://doi.org/10.1007/978-3-319-98720-0_47

History

- Fever, rigors
- Flank or abdominal pain
- Nausa, vomiting,
- Dysuria, UTI
- Weight loss, lethargy,
- Ileus, pleuritic pain or referred pain to the groin, thighs or knees

Examination

- Observations-Sats, RR, BP HR, Capillary refill time.
- Abdomen: flank tenderness (stones), flank mass, pelvic abcess, peritonitis.

Investigations

- A, B, C, D, E approach.
- IV lines.
- IV abx then fluids.
- Urine analysis/ culture-catheter and strict fluid balence.
- Bloods in FBC U+Es and clotting CRP, ABG.
- CT IVU.

Outcome

- If no blood dyscrasias, insert a percutaneous nephrostomy.
- Send off pus for culture from nephrostomy.
- ITU/ HDU care.
- IV antibiotics, usually Tazocin and Gentamicin.
- Give antibiotics according to culture sensitivity results.
- Strict fluid balence and resuscitation.
- (Meng et al)

Suggested Reading

Gardiner RA, Gwynne RA, Roberts SA. Perinephric abscess. BJU Int. 2011;107(Suppl 3):20–3.

Meng MV, Mario LA, McAninch JW. Current treatment and outcomes of perinephric abscesses. J Urol. 2002;168(4 Pt 1):1337–40.

Rubilotta E, Balzarro M, Lacola V, Sarti A, Porcaro AB, Artibani W. Current clinical management of renal and perinephric abscesses: a literature review. Urologia. 2014;81(3):144–7.

48 Diagnostic Pathway for Perinephric Abcess

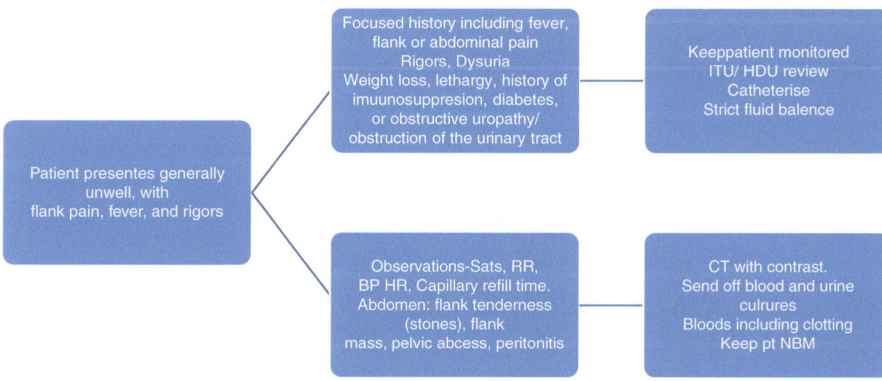

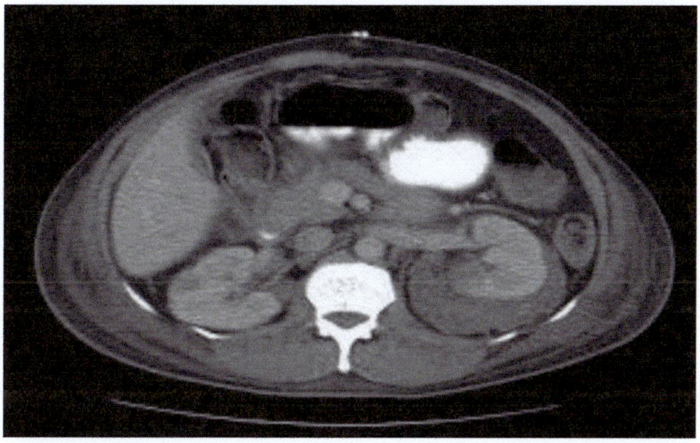

Fig. 48.1 CT demonstrating perinephric abcess

S. S. Goonewardene et al., *Basic Urological Management*,
https://doi.org/10.1007/978-3-319-98720-0_48

Suggested Reading

Gardiner RA, Gwynne RA, Roberts SA. Perinephric abscess. BJU Int. 2011;107(Suppl 3):20–3.

Meng MV, Mario LA, McAninch JW. Current treatment and outcomes of perinephric abscesses. J Urol. 2002;168(4 Pt 1):1337–40.

Rubilotta E, Balzarro M, Lacola V, Sarti A, Porcaro AB, Artibani W. Current clinical management of renal and perinephric abscesses: a literature review. Urologia. 2014;81(3):144–7.

Management Pathway for Perinephric Abcess

49

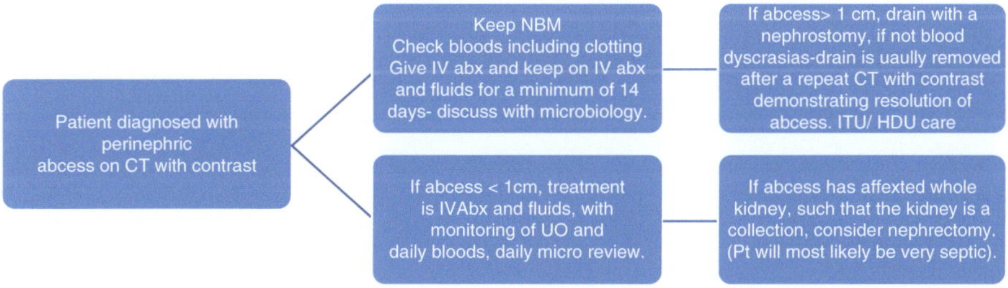

Suggested Reading

Gardiner RA, Gwynne RA, Roberts SA. Perinephric abscess. BJU Int. 2011;107(Suppl 3):20–3.

Meng MV, Mario LA, McAninch JW. Current treatment and outcomes of perinephric abscesses. J Urol. 2002;168(4 Pt 1):1337–40.

Rubilotta E, Balzarro M, Lacola V, Sarti A, Porcaro AB, Artibani W. Current clinical management of renal and perinephric abscesses: a literature review. Urologia. 2014;81(3):144–7.

S. S. Goonewardene et al., *Basic Urological Management*,
https://doi.org/10.1007/978-3-319-98720-0_49

50 Necrotising Fasciitis

Definition

- Infection of the skin and subcutaneous tissues.
- Life threatening-expedite surgical debridement.
- Spreads via the fascial planes.
- Commonly gas forming organisms
- Occurs often in diabetic patients.

Causes

- Risk factors: structurally abnormal urinary tract: diabetes, immunosupresion, smoking.
- Common organisms include Group A Streptococcus (group A strep), Klebsiella, Clostridium, Escherichia coli, Staphylococcus aureus, and Aeromonas hydrophila.
- Group A strep is considered the most common cause of necrotising fasciitis.

S. S. Goonewardene et al., *Basic Urological Management*,
https://doi.org/10.1007/978-3-319-98720-0_50

History

- Often starts as a small superficial infection area of infection but spreads within minutes.
- Tracks along the fascial planes.
- Fever, rigors,
- Acute onset, may have a history of minor trauma
- Urinary symptoms: LUTS, LTC, recurrent infections-prior history of infection and failed treatment with antibiotics.
- May have symptoms of being generally unwell.

Examination

- Abdomen and perineum:
  - Area of skin discolouration (mark area)
    - Necrosis
      - Crepitus (air beneath skin)
      - Palpable bladder
- Scrotal examination, review of external urethral meatus.

Investigations

- Simultaneous assessment and management
- Observations, if unstable, keep in A+E resusc and get ITU involved early
- A-sats (get oxygen on) B RR (nebs if required, mobile CXR), C-well perfused peripherally? peripheral pulses? or shut down?
- Lines in and IV fluids and abx-gentamicin, co-amoxiclav and metronidazole.
- Abdomen: flank tenderness (stones), palpable bladder (retention), ? bladder mass> CT.
- Look for other causes-rigid abdomen-? bowel perforation.
- Scrotal examination, review of external urethral meatus-examine for fournieres gangrene-catheterise.
- DRE: anal tone, sensation.

Outcome

- Keep patient NBM
- IVI access, IV abx-accoridng to trust policy-gent, metro and taz usually
- Fluid resuscitate and catheterise-strict fluid balence
- List for theatre-debridement, +/-stoma +/-orchidectomy
- (Inform General Sugery and Plastics for reconstruction or stoma, Inform microbiology for tissue sample from theatre).
- Anaesthetic assessment quickly and take patient to theatre
- (Czymek et al)

Suggested Reading

Czymek R, Kujath P, Bruch HP, Pfeiffer D, Nebrig M, Seehofer D, Guckelberger O. Treatment, outcome and quality of life after Fournier's gangrene: a multicentre study. Colorectal Dis. 2013;15(12):1529–36.

Polistena A, Cavallaro G, D'Ermo G, Avenia N, De Toma G. Fournier's gangrene: early diagnosis. How to diagnose, how to manage it. Minerva Chir. 2014;69(2):113–9.

Palvolgyi R, Kaji AH, Valeriano J, Plurad D, Rajfer J, de Virgilio C. Fournier's gangrene: a model for early prediction. Am Surg. 2014;80(10):926–31.

Shyam DC, Rapsang AG. Fournier's gangrene. Surgeon. 2013;11(4):222–32.

51 Diagnostic Pathway for Necrotising Fasciitis

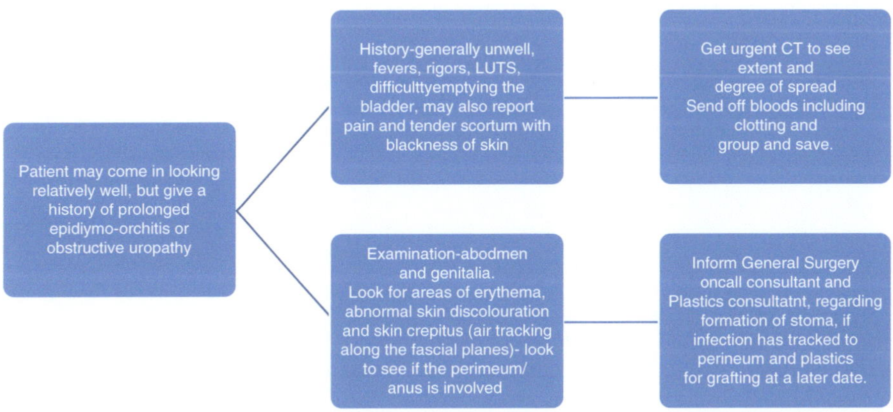

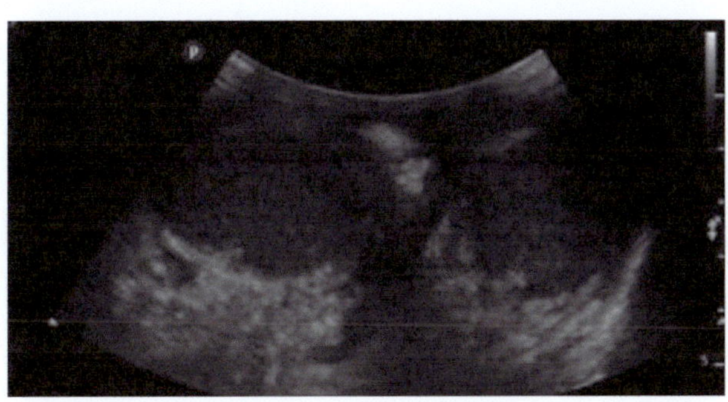

Fig. 51.1 USS demonstrating air within the scrotal tissues-necrotising fasciitis

S. S. Goonewardene et al., *Basic Urological Management*,
https://doi.org/10.1007/978-3-319-98720-0_51

Suggested Reading

Palvolgyi R, Kaji AH, Valeriano J, Plurad D, Rajfer J, de Virgilio C. Fournier's gangrene: a model for early prediction. Am Surg. 2014;80(10):926–31.
Polistena A, Cavallaro G, D'Ermo G, Avenia N, De Toma G. Fournier's gangrene: early diagnosis. How to diagnose, how to manage it. Minerva Chir. 2014;69(2):113–9.
Shyam DC, Rapsang AG. Fournier's gangrene. Surgeon. 2013;11(4):222–32.

52 Management Pathway for Necrotising Fasciitis

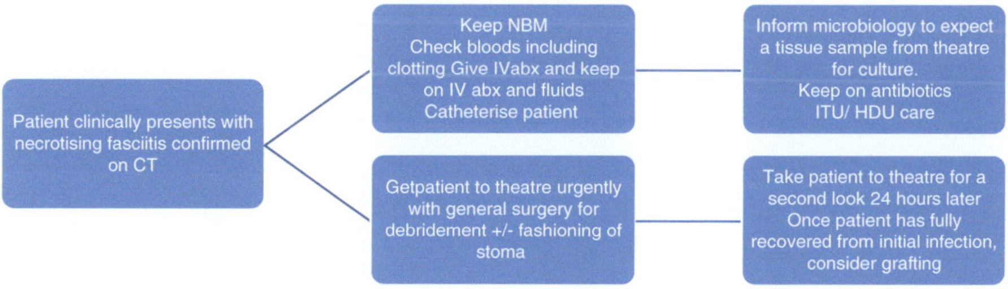

Suggested Reading

Czymek R, Kujath P, Bruch HP, Pfeiffer D, Nebrig M, Seehofer D, Guckelberger O. Treatment, outcome and quality of life after Fournier's gangrene: a multicentre study. Color Dis. 2013;15(12):1529–36.

S. S. Goonewardene et al., *Basic Urological Management*,
https://doi.org/10.1007/978-3-319-98720-0_52

53 Scrotal Abscess

Definition

- Collection of pus within the scrotum.
- Can be superficial and 'tent' the scrotal skin.
- Deep infections within the scrotum (testicular) can also result in deep seated abcess.
- Check for underlying testicular tumours (Arias -Cameron).
- It can also mimick torsion (Toh).

Causes

- Risk factors: structurally abnormal urinary tract: diabetes, immunosuppression, smoking.
- Epididymitis, if necrotising.
- Testicular abcess.
- Delayed torsion.
- Testicular Tumour.
- Patent processus vaginalis and appendicitis.

History

- Painful area, with no relief, often fluctuant having increased in size.
- Features of abcess: Callor-warmth, Rubor-redness, Dolor -pain, Tumour-mass.
- Fevers/ rigors/ LUTS/ UTIS.
- History of recurrent abcesses, or diabetes, post surgery.
- An USS is require for diagnosis (Miskin).

S. S. Goonewardene et al., *Basic Urological Management*,
https://doi.org/10.1007/978-3-319-98720-0_53

Examination

- Abdomen and perineum: area of skin discolouration (mark area),
- Erythema, swelling, redness present.
- Fluctuant lesion, tender to touch.
- Check no crepitus present (necrotising fasciitis)
- Assess the abdomen,? tender in RIF? appendicitis, palpable bladder?

Investigations

- Urine analysis and culture.
- Bloods: FBS, clotting renal function and LFTS.
- Pus swab if abcess burst.

Outcome

- Keep patient NBM, give IV abx.
- Take patient to theater for incision and drainage of abcess.
- Use a yates drain to keep the abcess open-remove on the ward the next day.
- Scrotal abcesses are superficial and do not normally require packing.

Suggested Reading

Arias-Camison JM, Desilva HN, Panthagani I, Twohig MT, Bourque MD. Scrotal abcess mimicking testicular torsion in a premature infant. Conn Med. 2009;73(4):215–6.

Miskin M, Buckspan M, Bain J. Ultrasonographic examination of scrotal masses. J Urol. 1977;117(2):185–8.

Toh JW, Gibson K, Vanlioglu B, Ang S, Ong E. Rapid progression of perianal abscess into Fournier's gangrene. ANZ J Surg. 2015;85(3):192–3.

Diagnostic Pathway for Scrotal Abcess

54

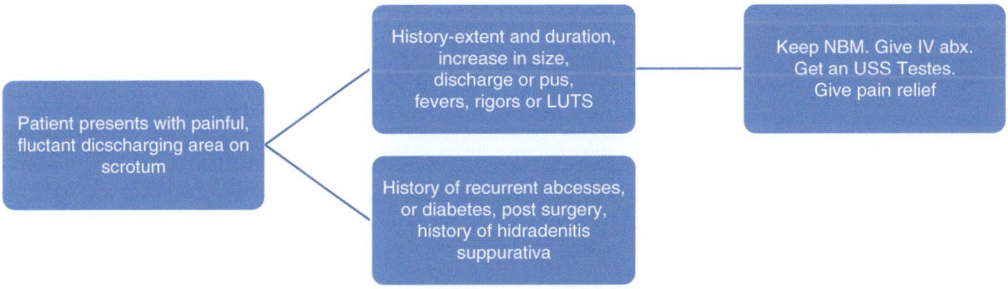

Fig. 54.1 Demonstrating an USS of the scrotum with a scrotal abcess

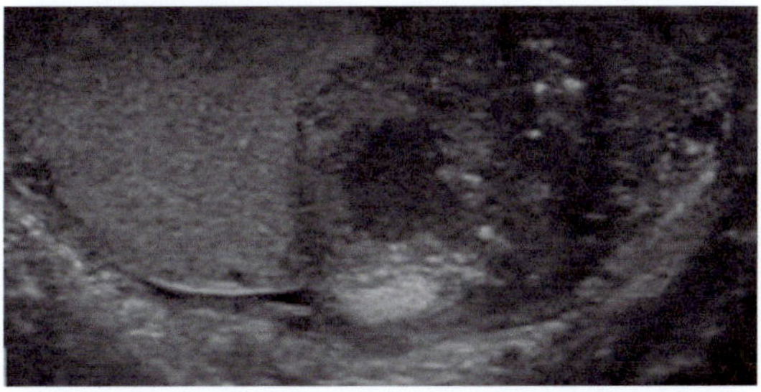

Suggested Reading

Arias-Camison JM, Desilva HN, Panthagani I, Twohig MT, Bourque MD. Scrotal abcess mimicking testicular torsion in a premature infant. Conn Med. 2009;73(4):215–6.

Miskin M, Buckspan M, Bain J. Ultrasonographic examination of scrotal masses. J Urol. 1977;117(2):185–8.

Toh JW, Gibson K, Vanlioglu B, Ang S, Ong E. Rapid progression of perianal abscess into Fournier's gangrene. ANZ J Surg. 2015;85(3):192–3.

S. S. Goonewardene et al., *Basic Urological Management*,
https://doi.org/10.1007/978-3-319-98720-0_54

55 Management Pathway for Scrotal Abcess

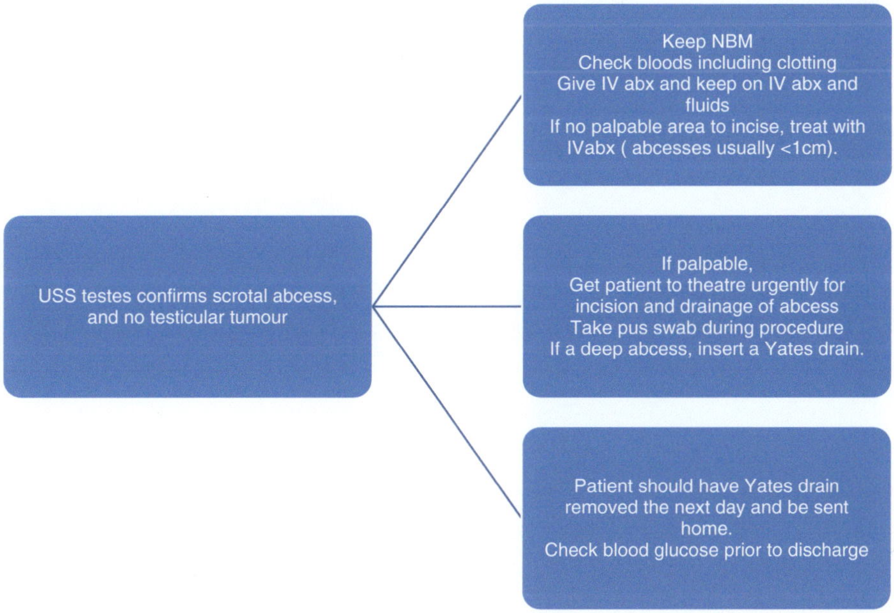

S. S. Goonewardene et al., *Basic Urological Management*,
https://doi.org/10.1007/978-3-319-98720-0_55

Epididymitis/Orchitis

56

Definition

- Infection within the scrotum result in inflammation of the epididiymis, testicle or both together.
- This can be acute, chronic or acute on chronic.
- Acutely painful when it does occur.
- In patients with a painful testicle < 20 years, rule out torsion with surgical exploration.

Causes

- In sexually active: chlamydia, gonnorrhoea or E.Coli.
- Urinary tract organisms: E.coli, Proteus, Klebsiella.
- Post operation: cystocopy, prostatectomy, vasectomy.
- Inflammatory non infectious causes: reflux of urine, chemical epididymitis-amiodarone.
- Post catheterisation.
- Differentials: testicular torsion, testicular tumour, hernia, lipoma of the cord, hydrocoele
- (Stewart et al)

S. S. Goonewardene et al., *Basic Urological Management*,
https://doi.org/10.1007/978-3-319-98720-0_56

History

- Painful, red, hot swollen testicle.
- May have an associated UTI or LUTS with incomplete emptying.
- Gradual onset of pain, developing over days.
- Check for LTC.
- Associated frequency and urgency.
- Urethral discharge.
- History of recurrent infection, or diabetes, post surgery or catherisation.
- (Naber et al)

Examination

- Abdomen and perineum: check for fourniers gangene-area of skin discolouration (mark area), necrosis, crepitus (air beneath skin).
- Scrotal skin change in longstanding cases-induration, tenting of skin (abcess), localised fluctuant area (infected sebaceous cyst).
- Scrotal examination, review of external urethral meatus-red hot swollen testicle, normal lye, non high riding. cremasteric reflex present.

Investigations

- Simultaneous assessment and management
- Urine culture.
- If septic, blood cultures.
- IV line access.
- Bloods: FBC, CRP, Renal function.
- USS scrotum-to rule out abcess or tumour.
- (Hebener et al)

Outcome

- IVI access, IV abx-accoridng to trust policy-gent, metro and taz usually.
- Fluid resuscitate and catheterise-strict fluid balence.
- Treat with antibiotics for 14 days, give a scrotal support.
- If severe and changed to fourniers gangrene, resuscitate and list for debridement +/– stoma +/– orchidectomy in theatre.

Suggested Reading

Herbener TE. Ultrasound in the assessment of the acute scrotum. J Clin Ultrasound. 1996;24(8):405–21.

Naber KG, Bergman B, Bishop MC, Bjerklund-Johansen TE, Botto H, Lobel B, Jinenez Cruz F, Selvaggi FP. EAU guidelines for the management of urinary and male genital tract infections. Urinary Tract Infection (UTI) Working Group of the Health Care Office (HCO) of the European Association of Urology (EAU). Eur Urol. 2001;40(5):576–88.

Stewart A, Ubee SS, Davies H. Epididymo-orchitis. BMJ. 2011;342:d1543.

57 Diagnostic Pathway for Epididymo-Orchitis

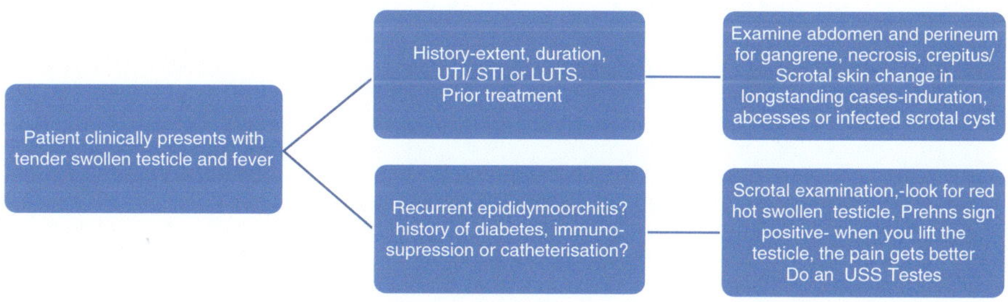

Suggested Reading

Herbener TE. Ultrasound in the assessment of the acute scrotum. J Clin Ultrasound. 1996;24(8):405–21.

Naber KG, Bergman B, Bishop MC, Bjerklund-Johansen TE, Botto H, Lobel B, Jinenez Cruz F, Selvaggi FP. EAU guidelines for the management of urinary and male genital tract infections. Urinary Tract Infection (UTI) Working Group of the Health Care Office (HCO) of the European Association of Urology (EAU). Eur Urol. 2001;40(5):576–88.

Stewart A, Ubee SS, Davies H. Epididymo-orchitis. BMJ. 2011;342:d1543.

S. S. Goonewardene et al., *Basic Urological Management*, https://doi.org/10.1007/978-3-319-98720-0_57

58 Management Pathway for Epididymo-Orchtis

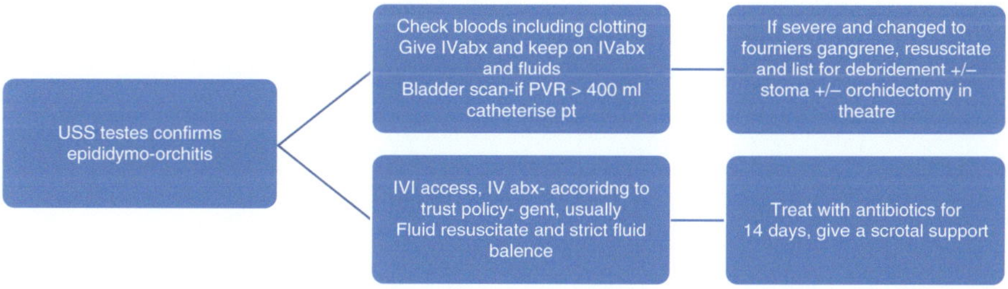

Suggested Reading

Herbener TE. Ultrasound in the assessment of the acute scrotum. J Clin Ultrasound. 1996;24(8):405–21.

Naber KG, Bergman B, Bishop MC, Bjerklund-Johansen TE, Botto H, Lobel B, Jinenez Cruz F, Selvaggi FP. EAU guidelines for the management of urinary and male genital tract infections. Urinary Tract Infection (UTI) Working Group of the Health Care Office (HCO) of the European Association of Urology (EAU). Eur Urol. 2001;40(5):576–88.

Stewart A, Ubee SS, Davies H. Epididymo-orchitis. BMJ. 2011;342:d1543.

S. S. Goonewardene et al., *Basic Urological Management*,
https://doi.org/10.1007/978-3-319-98720-0_58

59 Prostatitis

Definition

- Inflammation within the prostate.
- It can be infectious or non infectious.
- It may be acute or chronic.
- The condition is acutely painful and persistent and can be associated with chronic pelvic pain (Engeler et al).

Causes

- Incomplete emptying of the bladder and LUTS.
- Urinary tract organisms: E.coli, Proteus, Klebsiella.
- Post operation: vasectomy.
- Prostatic calculi.
- Post catheterisation.
- Differentials: testicular torsion, testicular tumour, hernia, lipoma of the cord, hydrocoele.

S. S. Goonewardene et al., *Basic Urological Management*,
https://doi.org/10.1007/978-3-319-98720-0_59

History

- LUTS (obstructive), incomplete emptying, UTIs.
- Perineal pain-acute and persistent, low back or pelvic pain.
- Recurrent UTIS.
- Dysuria, prostatic calculic being passes, urethral discharge.
- Fever, chills, myalgia, arthralgia, premature ejaculation, pain on ejaculation.
- History of being post sclerotherapy for rectal cancer.
- (Dickinson)

Examination

- Abdomen and perineum: Palpable bladder (incomplete emptying), tenderness in flanks (retention)
- Scrotal skin changes
- Tender perineum
- DRE: size, tenderness (prostatitis/ abcess), consistency of prostate (boggy prostate, abcess).

Investigations

- Urine culture (DRE then collection of urine culture).
- If septic, blood cultures
- IV line
- Bloods: FBC, CRP, Renal function
- TRUS/MRI to rule out abcess.
- PSA later

Outcome

- IVI access, IV abx- accoridng to trust policy- gent, metro and taz usually.
- Fluid resuscitate and catheterise- strict fluid balence.
- Treat with antibiotics.
- Even if abcess, consider IV antibiotic therapy 1st. Drainage of a prostatic abcess can make a patent septic enough to require ITU.
- NSAIDS and tamsulosin.
- Lifestyle measures- avoid stress, try and identify triggers.
- Physical therapy, massage therapy, exercise therapy.
- Sepsis source control.
- Prevention: drink 1.5 L water a day.
- (Rees et al)

Suggested Reading

Dickson G. Prostatitis—diagnosis and treatment. Aust Fam Physician. 2013;42(4):216.

Rees J, Abrahams M, Doble A, Cooper A, Prostatitis Expert Reference Group (PERG). Diagnosis and treatment of chronic bacterial prostatitis and chronic prostatitis/chronic pelvic pain syndrome: a consensus guideline. BJU Int. 2015;116(4):509–25.

Wagenlehner FM, Pilatz A, Bschleipfer T, Diemer T, Linn T, Meinhardt A, Schagdarsurengin U. Bacterial prostatitis. World J Urol. 2013;31(4):711–6.

60 Diagnostic Pathway for Prostatitis

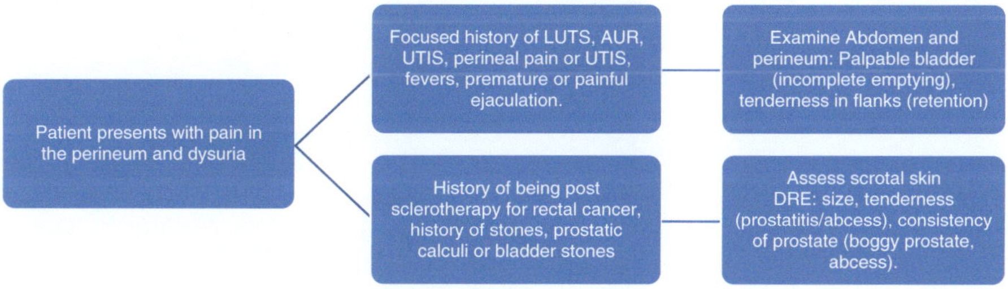

S. S. Goonewardene et al., *Basic Urological Management*,
https://doi.org/10.1007/978-3-319-98720-0_60

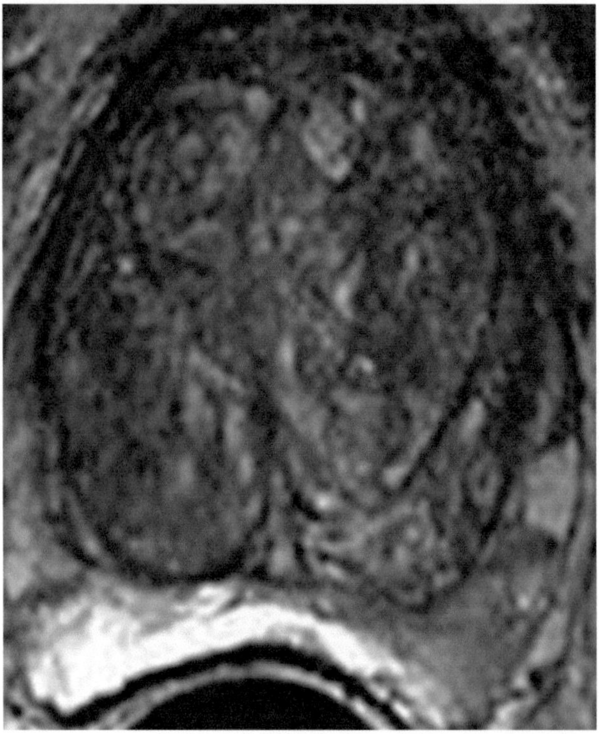

Fig. 60.1 MRI demonstrating acute prostatitis

Suggested Reading

Dickson G. Prostatitis—diagnosis and treatment. Aust Fam Physician. 2013;42(4):216.

Rees J, Abrahams M, Doble A, Cooper A, Prostatitis Expert Reference Group (PERG). Diagnosis and treatment of chronic bacterial prostatitis and chronic prostatitis/chronic pelvic pain syndrome: a consensus guideline. BJU Int. 2015;116(4):509–25.

Wagenlehner FM, Pilatz A, Bschleipfer T, Diemer T, Linn T, Meinhardt A, Schagdarsurengin U. Bacterial prostatitis. World J Urol. 2013;31(4):711–6.

Management Pathway for Prostatitis

61

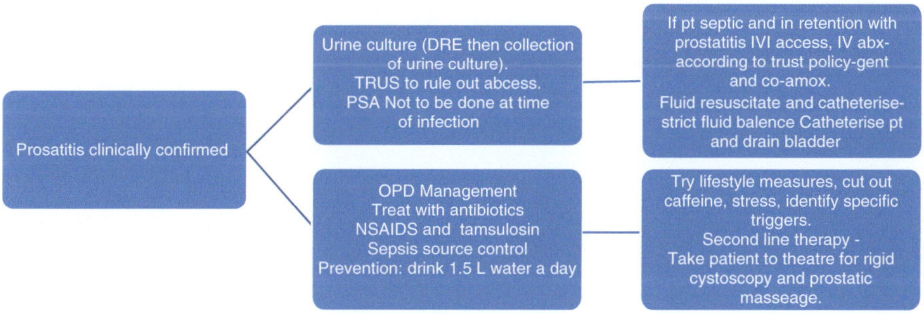

Suggested Reading

Dickson G. Prostatitis—diagnosis and treatment. Aust Fam Physician. 2013;42(4):216.

Rees J, Abrahams M, Doble A, Cooper A, Prostatitis Expert Reference Group (PERG). Diagnosis and treatment of chronic bacterial prostatitis and chronic prostatitis/chronic pelvic pain syndrome: a consensus guideline. BJU Int. 2015;116(4):509–25.

Wagenlehner FM, Pilatz A, Bschleipfer T, Diemer T, Linn T, Meinhardt A, Schagdarsurengin U. Bacterial prostatitis. World J Urol. 2013;31(4):711–6.

S. S. Goonewardene et al., *Basic Urological Management*,
https://doi.org/10.1007/978-3-319-98720-0_61

62 Renal/Ureteric Colic

Definition

- Caused by renal calculi passing through the urinary tract, causing obstruction to the flow of urine.
- Pain is acute, usually in the flanks radiatng to groin.
- Pain does not improve, no matter what position the patient is in.
- Intermittent pain (colicky) which becomes persistent.
- (Teichman et al)

Causes

- Risk factors for stones:
- Decreased water intake < 1.5L.
- Caffeine intake.
- High protein or salt diet.
- Vitamin supplements.
- Diet high in broccoli or spinach (Calcium oxalate).
- High consumption of dairy products.
- Urinary tract infections, poor urinary drainage.
- (Turk et al).

S. S. Goonewardene et al., *Basic Urological Management*,
https://doi.org/10.1007/978-3-319-98720-0_62

History

- Flank pain-radiating to groin (if stone is passing).
- Fever, chills, rigors.
- Nausea and vomiting.
- Luts and prior obstruction.
- Haematuria.
- Prior history of stones, operations, stent insertion.
- Risk factors for stones (box above)

Examination

- Observations- is the patient pyrexial or septi?
- Abdomen: Tenderness in flanks, radiating to groin, palpable mass in flanks (?renal tumour/clot colic), palpable bladder (retention, stones obstructing).
- Rule out other pathology- AAA, acute appendicitis, bowel perforation, chest infection, ovarian cyst, ileus.
- Scrotal examination, review of external urethral meatus (? tight-phimosis/BXO), passage of any stones in urine- has the patient passed it out?

Investigations

- Urine analysis and culture- catheterise if septic.
- If septic, blood cultures, ABG.
- IV lines.
- Bloods: FBC, CRP, Renal function.
- In a septic patient, simultaneous assessment and management.
- CT KUB- plain CT- low dose.
- Do not do a CT with contrast as stones will not be seen. (stones are white on CT, contrast is also white).

Outcome

- IVI access, IV abx- accoridng to trust policy- gentamicin usuall. Even if renal; function deranged- giveone renal dose of gent and discuss with microbiology re policy- co-amoxiclav if not penicillin allergic.
- Fluid resuscitate and catheterise- strict fluid balence.
- Treat with antibiotics, check sensitivitites on blood and urine culture.
- NSAIDS and tamsulosin- if stone < 5mm, in ureter with no evidence of obstruction, hydronephrosis or perinephric stranding, normal renal function, no sepsis.
- If evidence of obstuction, stone 6mm or greater, deranged renal function-patient requires rigid cystioscopy and ureteric stents.
- If patient septic with obstructive stone, for neprostomy insertion with antegrade stents and nephrostomyremoval at a later date.
- ITU/ HDU admission if eptic and HD unstable.
- Follow-up: Stone clinic to preassess patient. If stone < 1 cm none obstructive For ESWL.. If stented and < 1 cm for URS. If > 1 cm and in renal pelvis for PCNL.
- (Bultitude et al)

Suggested Reading

Bultitude M, Rees J. Management of renal colic. Eur Urol. 2016;69(3):468–74.

Teichman JM. Clinical practice. Acute renal colic from ureteral calculus. N Engl J Med. 2004;350(7):684–93.

Türk C, Petřík A, Sarica K, Seitz C, Skolarikos A, Straub M, Knoll T. EAU guidelines on diagnosis and conservative management of urolithiasis. Eur Urol. 2016;69(3):468–74.

63 Diagnostic Pathway for Stones

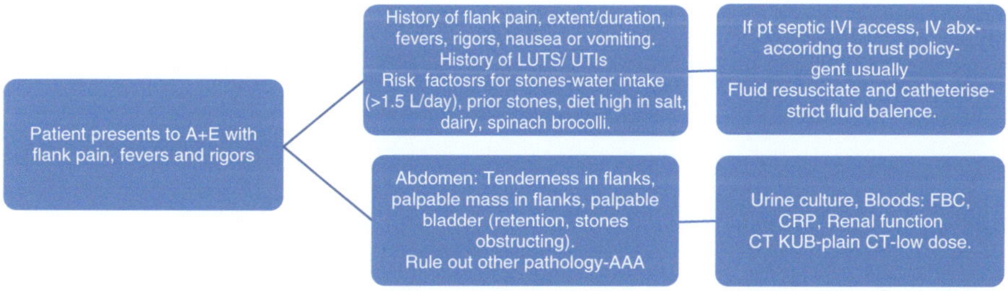

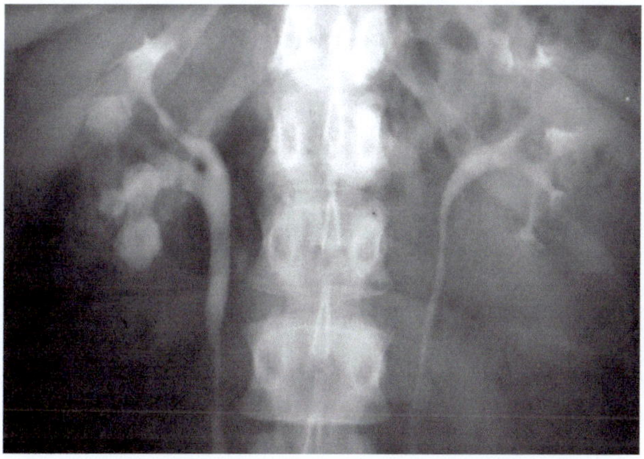

Fig. 63.1 An IVU (intravenous urogram)

S. S. Goonewardene et al., *Basic Urological Management*,
https://doi.org/10.1007/978-3-319-98720-0_63

Suggested Reading

Bultitude M, Rees J. Management of renal colic. Eur Urol. 2016;69(3):468–74.

Teichman JM. Clinical practice. Acute renal colic from ureteral calculus. N Engl J Med. 2004;350(7):684–93.

Türk C, Petřík A, Sarica K, Seitz C, Skolarikos A, Straub M, Knoll T. EAU guidelines on diagnosis and conservative management of urolithiasis. Eur Urol. 2016;69(3):468–74.

64 Management Pathway for Renal Stones

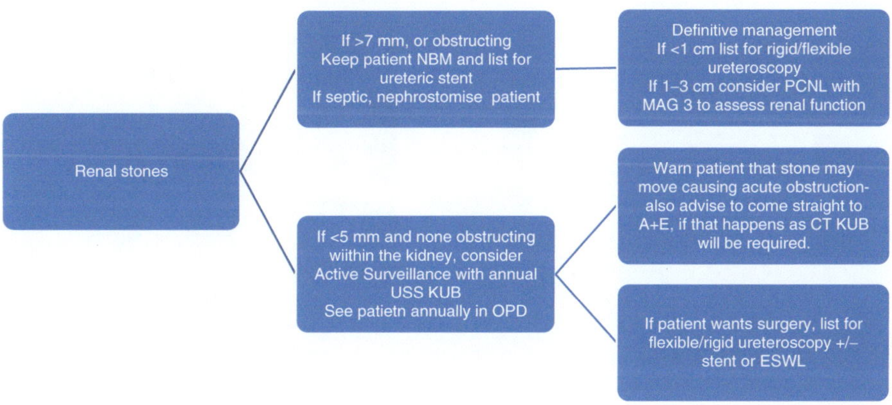

S. S. Goonewardene et al., *Basic Urological Management*,
https://doi.org/10.1007/978-3-319-98720-0_64

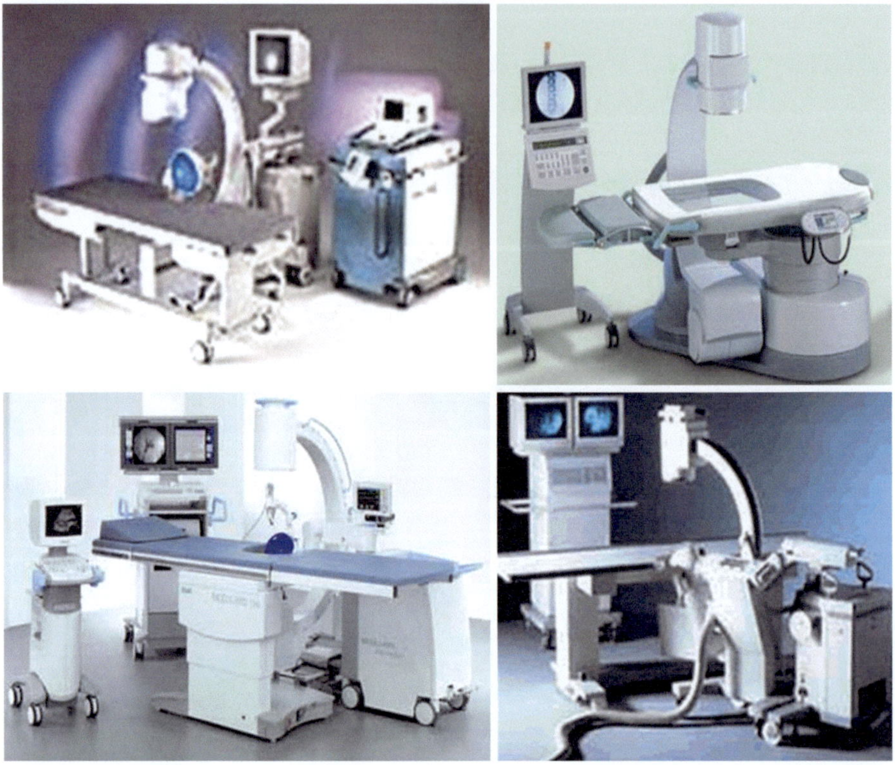

Fig. 64.1 New generation lithotripters for ESWL

Fig. 64.2 Appearance of ureter at ureteroscopy with guidewire

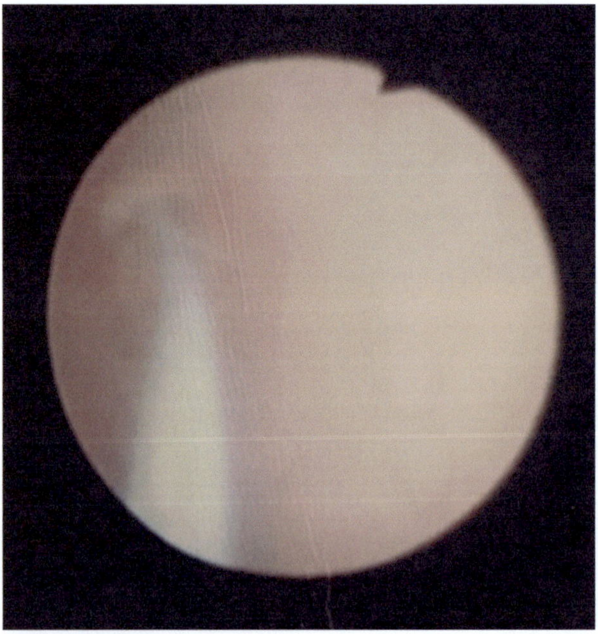

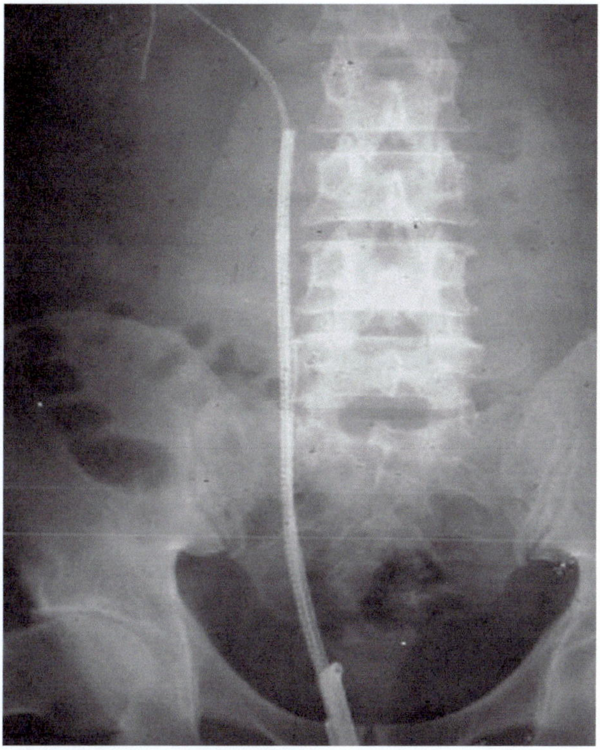

Fig. 64.3 Passage of a flexible ureteroscope over a guide wire to the right kidney

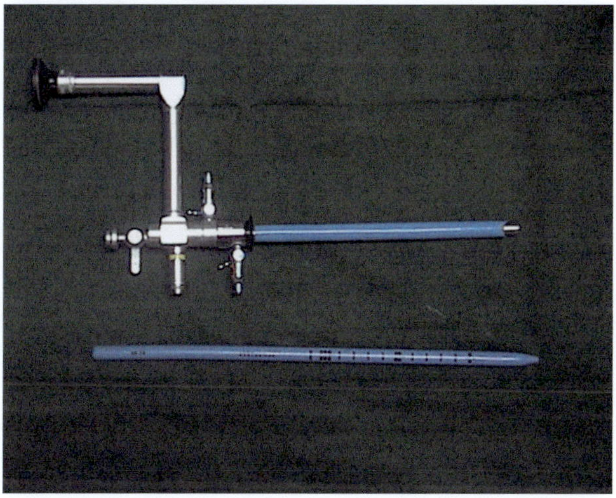

Fig. 64.4 A nephroscope for PCNL and dilators for insertion

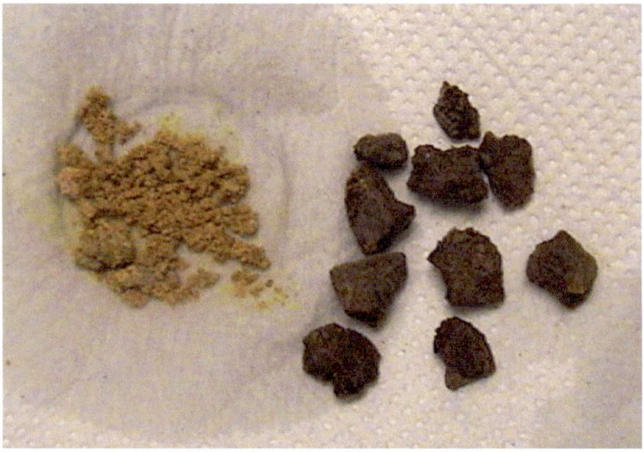

Fig. 64.5 Renal stones extracted at PCNL

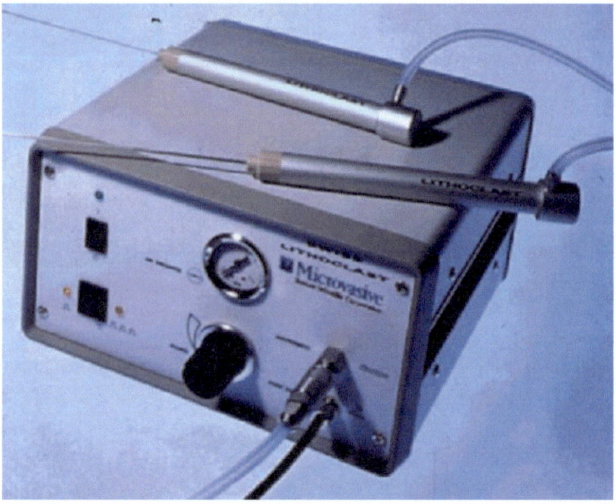

Fig. 64.6 The intracorporeal lithotripter for stone extraction

Suggested Reading

Bultitude M, Rees J. Management of renal colic. Eur Urol. 2016;69(3):468–74.

Teichman JM. Clinical practice. Acute renal colic from ureteral calculus. N Engl J Med. 2004;350(7):684–93.

Türk C, Petřík A, Sarica K, Seitz C, Skolarikos A, Straub M, Knoll T. EAU guidelines on diagnosis and conservative management of urolithiasis. Eur Urol. 2016;69(3):468–74.

65 Management Pathway for Ureteric Stones

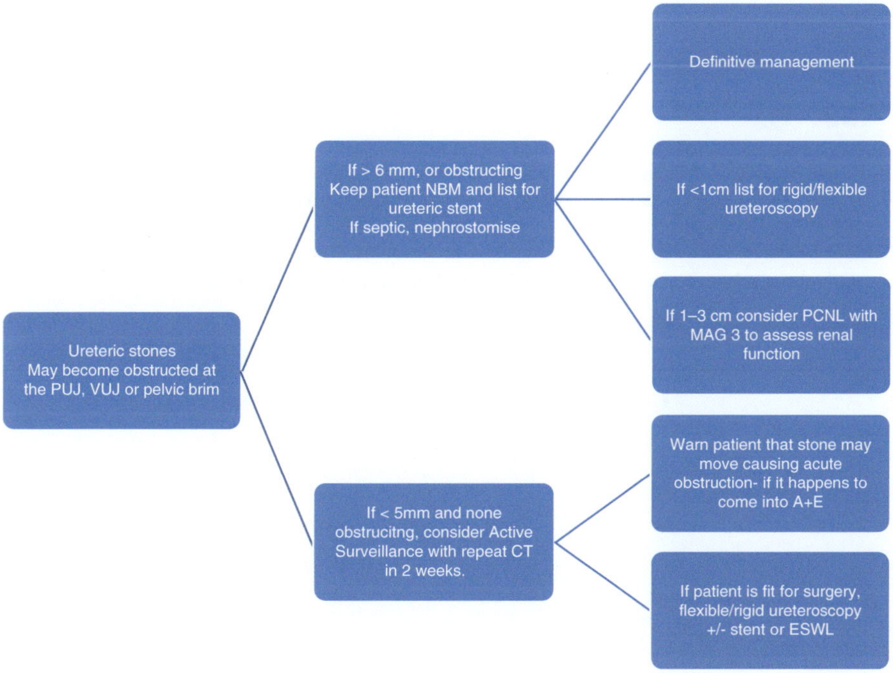

S. S. Goonewardene et al., *Basic Urological Management*,
https://doi.org/10.1007/978-3-319-98720-0_65

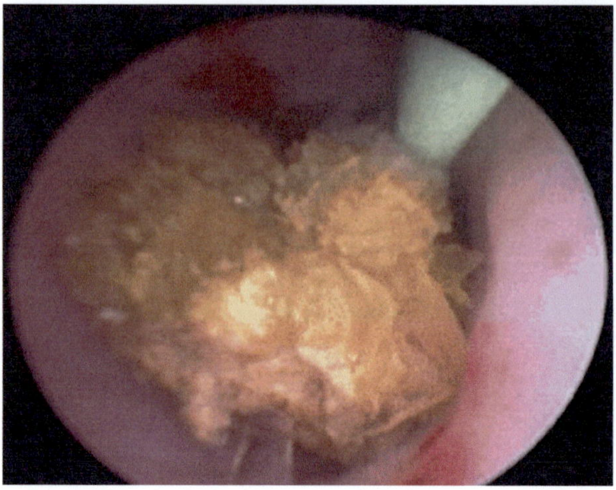

Fig. 65.1 Laser fragementation of stone in ureter. The laster is seen at 6 o'clock and the guidewire appears green (PTFE) at 1 o'clock

Suggested Reading

Bultitude M, Rees J. Management of renal colic. Eur Urol. 2016;69(3):468–74.

Teichman JM. Clinical practice. Acute renal colic from ureteral calculus. N Engl J Med. 2004;350(7):684–93.

Türk C, Petřík A, Sarica K, Seitz C, Skolarikos A, Straub M, Knoll T. EAU guidelines on diagnosis and conservative management of urolithiasis. Eur Urol. 2016;69(3):468–74.

66 Ureteral Clot Colic

Definition

- Colic caused by blood clot passing from the kidney or renal pelvis down the ureter to the bladder
- The pain is caused by the clot obstructing the ureter.
- The origin of the blood clot is most often from RCC of the kidney, or TCC of the urothelium.
- If obstructed for a period of time, patients can present with sepsis.

Causes

- Bleeding and clots in the urinary tract (ureter).
- Renal cell carcinoma of the kidney.
- Transitional cell carcinoma of the urothelium.
- Urinary tract infection.
- Renal or ureteric stones.
- Post operative-partal/nephrectomy, pyeloplasty, post ureteric stent insertion.
- Bleeding diathesis, haemophilia. (Evins et al)
- Henoch Schlon Purpura leading to urethritis (Robson et al)

History

- Flank pain-radiating to groin (as clot passes).
- Fever, chills, rigors.
- Nausea and vomiting.
- Haematuria-look for histroy of prior haematuria investigations.
- Prior history of stones, operations, stent insertion.
- Risk factors for stones (box above)/Pain.

S. S. Goonewardene et al., *Basic Urological Management*,
https://doi.org/10.1007/978-3-319-98720-0_66

Suggested Reading

Evins SC, McInnes BK. Ureteral colic secondary to blood clot in hemophiliac. Urology. 1979;13(6):650–1.

Robson WL, Leung AK, Mathers MS, Robson WL, Leung AK, Mathers MS. Renal colic due to Henoch-Schönlein purpura. J S C Med Assoc. 1994;90(12):592–5.

Tanriverdi O, Yencilek F, Koyuncu H, Yencilek E, Sarica K. Emergent stenting after uncomplicated ureteroscopy: evaluation of 23 patients. Urology. 2011;77(2):305–8.

67 Diagnosis of Ureteral Clot Colic

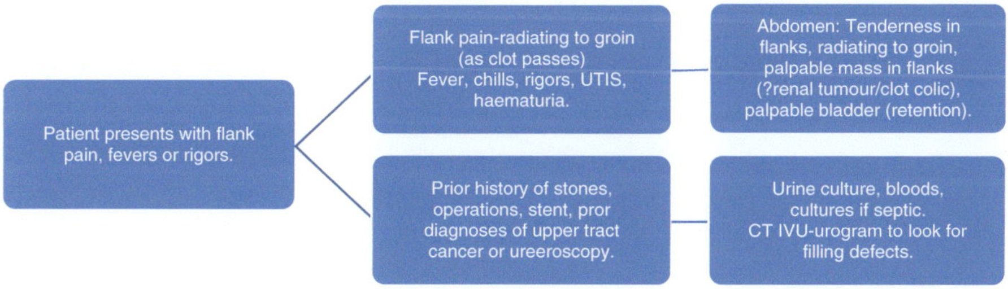

Suggested Reading

Evins SC, McInnes BK. Ureteral colic secondary to blood clot in hemophiliac. Urology. 1979;13(6):650–1.

Robson WL, Leung AK, Mathers MS, Robson WL, Leung AK, Mathers MS. Renal colic due to Henoch-Schönlein purpura. J S C Med Assoc. 1994;90(12):592–5.

Tanriverdi O, Yencilek F, Koyuncu H, Yencilek E, Sarica K. Emergent stenting after uncomplicated ureteroscopy: evaluation of 23 patients. Urology. 2011;77(2):305–8.

S. S. Goonewardene et al., *Basic Urological Management*,
https://doi.org/10.1007/978-3-319-98720-0_67

Management of Ureteral Clot Colic

68

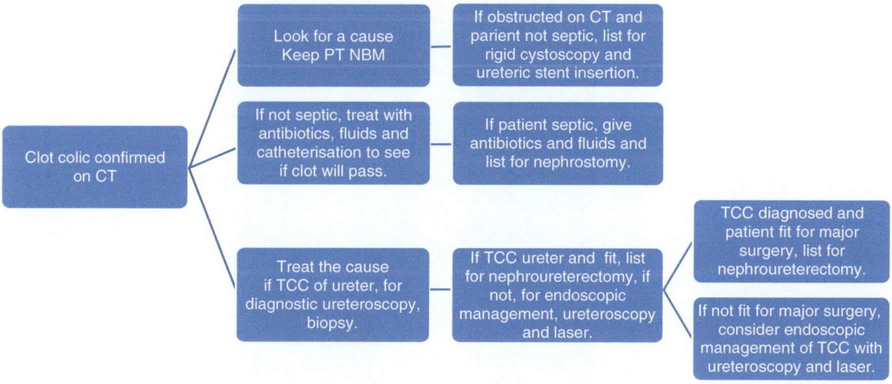

S. S. Goonewardene et al., *Basic Urological Management*,
https://doi.org/10.1007/978-3-319-98720-0_68

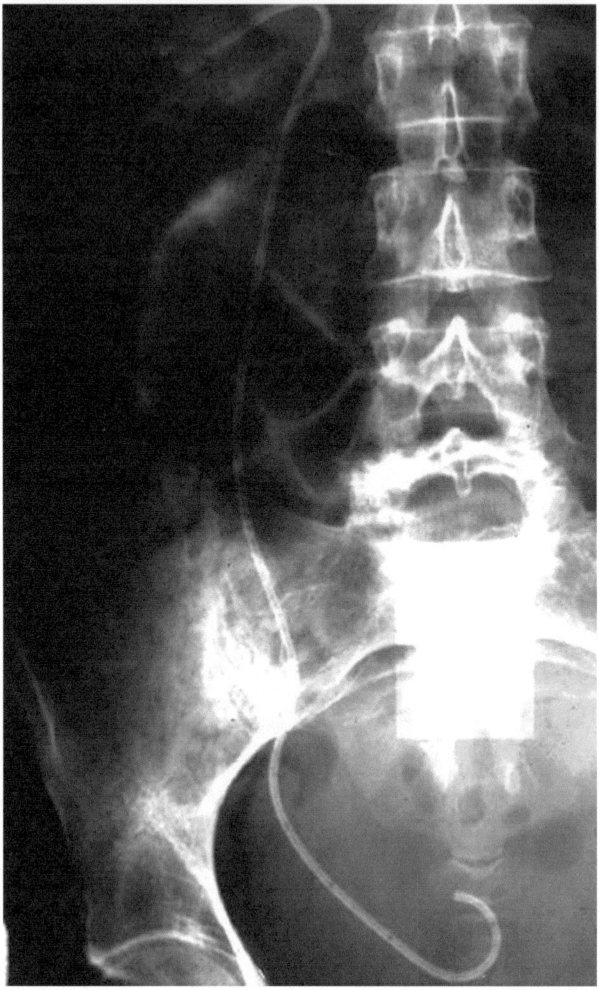

Fig. 68.1 Stent in situ with extravasation

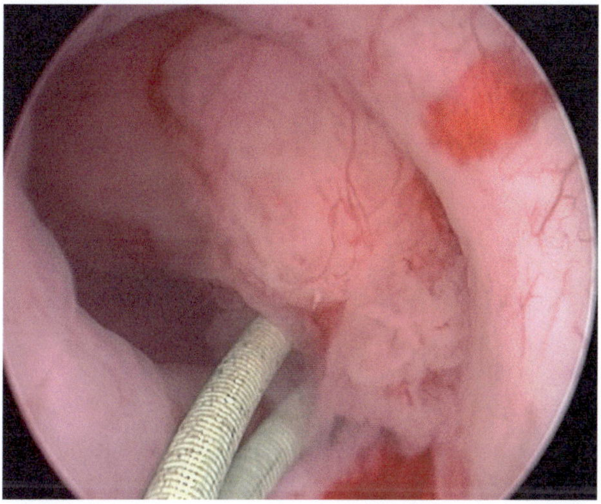

Fig. 68.2 TCC tumour in ureter

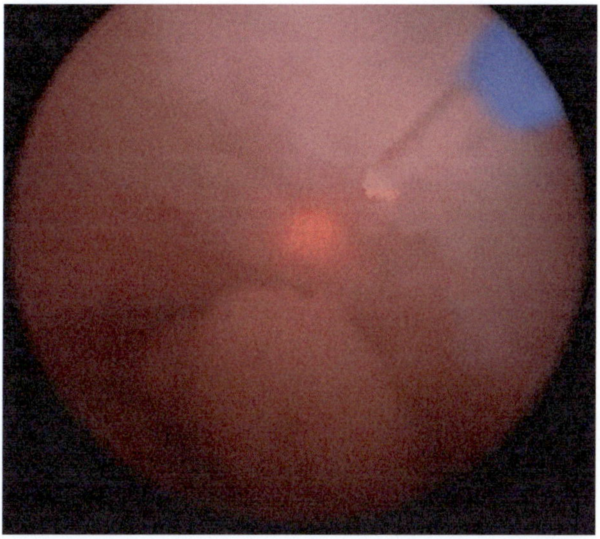

Fig. 68.3 Laser fulguration of TCC ureter

Suggested Reading

Evins SC, McInnes BK. Ureteral colic secondary to blood clot in hemophiliac. Urology. 1979;13(6):650–1.

Robson WL, Leung AK, Mathers MS, Robson WL, Leung AK, Mathers MS. Renal colic due to Henoch-Schönlein purpura. J S C Med Assoc. 1994;90(12):592–5.

Tanriverdi O, Yencilek F, Koyuncu H, Yencilek E, Sarica K. Emergent stenting after uncomplicated ureteroscopy: evaluation of 23 patients. Urology. 2011;77(2):305–8.

Pelvi-Ureteric Junction Obstruction

69

Definition

- Narrowing of the ureter where it joins the renal pelvis.
- The pain is caused by impaired flow of urine.
- This type of obstruction can also impair renal function.
- Whilst a CT urogram (with contrast) will delineate anatomy, a MAG 3 renogram with post micturition phase will be diagnostic of obstruction.
- Most often, the patient presents to OPD with intermittent niggling pain, but this patient can also present septic in obstruction.

Causes

- Congenital.
- One of the most common causes of hydronephrosis in children.
- It can also arise in the lower pole moiety of duplex systems or incomplete duplex systems (Avlan et al, Gonzalez et al).
- There is a familial association to those suffering from Vescio ureteric reflux (Manouvrier et al).
- It can be associated with bilateral multicystic dysplasia (Groener).

S. S. Goonewardene et al., *Basic Urological Management*,
https://doi.org/10.1007/978-3-319-98720-0_69

History

- Intermittent flank pain (Ward).
- Recurrent UTIS or stones (Atug et al, Wah et al).
- Worse at night, after drining large amounts of fluid or alcohol.
- Fevers and rigors, sepsis.
- Presentation with pyonephrosis.
- LUTS.

Examination

- Abdomen: Tenderness in flanks, radiating to groin, palpable mass in flanks (?renal tumour/clot colic), palpable bladder (retention).
- Rule out other pathology- AAA, acute appendicitis, bowel perforation, chest infection, ovarian cyst, ileus.

Investigations

- Urine analysis and culture- catheterise if septic
- Uroflowmetry and post void residual (ensure the patient is not in retention and emptying properly.
- Bloods- renal function, FBC and CRP.
- CT urogram to see anatomy and MAG 3 renogram with post micturition (Tasca et al).

Outcome

- If patient has PJUO wth impairment of renal function, and is fit for procedure-counsel regarding pyeloplasty- lap or robotic.
- Follow-up MAG 3 renogram to reassess split renal function and blood to asessrenal function.
- Patients can be conservatively managed if renal function is stable, but they need to be very closely followed up (Goyal et al).
- However, if a patient is symptomatic, septic or has deranged renal function emergency intervention is needed.
- In the first instance, this would be a stent or nephrostomy, but definitive therapy would be a pyeloplasty.
- This can be done via endoscopic, open, laparoscopic or robotic methods.
- If unfit for major surgery, it can be managed with regular stent changes.

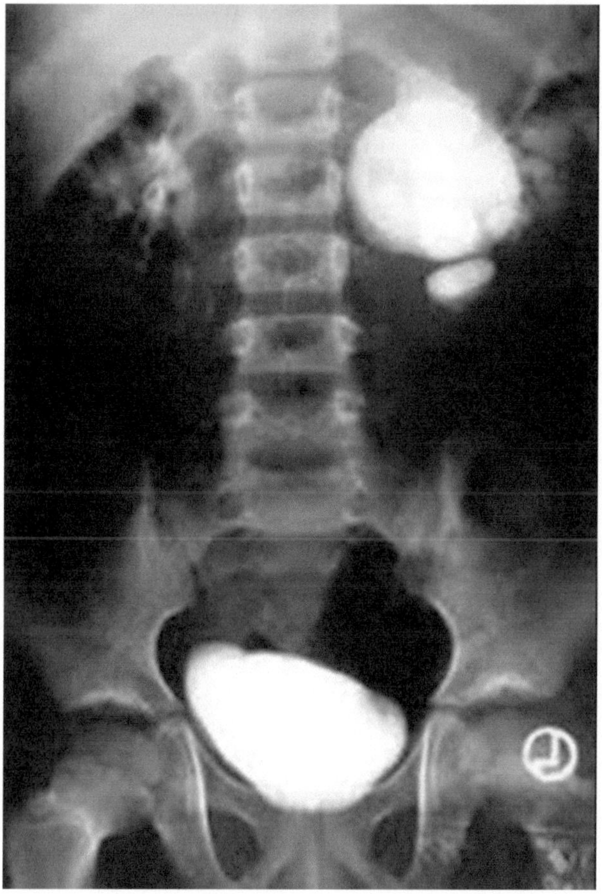

Fig. 69.1 IVU demonstrating PUJO

Suggested Reading

Atug F, Castle EP, Burgess SV, Thomas R. Concomitant management of renal calculi and pelvi-ureteric junction obstruction with robotic laparoscopic surgery. BJU Int. 2005;96(9):1365–8.

Avlan D, Gündoğdu G, Delibaş A, Nayci A. Pyeloureterostomy in the management of the lower pole pelvi-ureteric junction obstruction in incomplete duplicated systems. Urology. 2010;76(6):1468–71.

Gonzalez F, Canning DA, Hyun G, Casale P. Lower pole pelvi-ureteric junction obstruction in duplicated collecting systems. BJU Int. 2006;97(1):161–5.

Goyal NK, Goel A, Yadav R. Conservative management of pelvi-ureteric junction obstruction (PUJO): is it appropriate and if so what duration of follow-up is needed? BJU Int. 2012;110(1):E1.

Groenen PM, Vanderlinden G, Devriendt K, Fryns JP, Van de Ven WJ. Rearrangement of the human CDC5L gene by a t(6;19)(p21;q13.1) in a patient with multicystic renal dysplasia. Genomics. 1998;49(2):218–29.

Manouvrier-Hanu S, Devisme L, Farre I, Hue V, Storme L, Kacet N, Boute-Benejean O, Farriaux JP. Pulmonary hypertension of the newborn and urogenital anomalies in two male siblings: a new family with misalignment of pulmonary vessels. Genet Couns. 1996;7(4):249–55.

Tasca A, Barulli M, Artibani W, Passerini G, Bui F, Cagnato P, Macri C. Role of the diuresis renogram in the study of the pelviureteric junction. Eur Urol. 1985;11(6):374–7.

Wah TM, Weston MJ, Irving HC. Lower moiety pelvic-ureteric junction obstruction (PUJO) of the duplex kidney presenting with pyonephrosis in adults. Br J Radiol. 2003;76(912):909–12.

Ward HC, Brereton RJ. Pelviureteric junction obstruction and recurrent abdominal pain in childhood. Br J Surg. 1989;76(8):818–9.

Diagnosis of PUJO

70

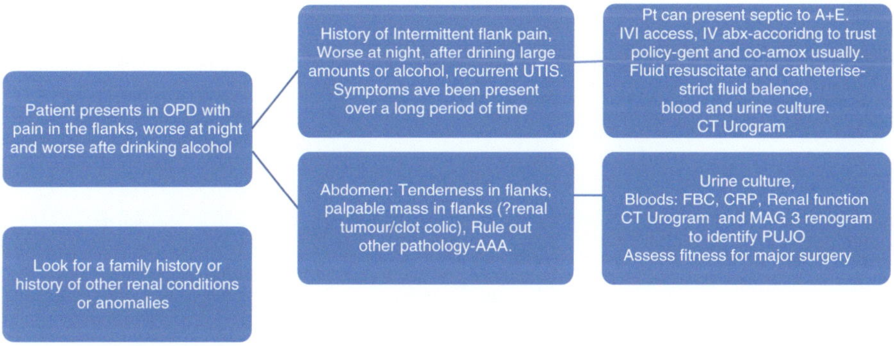

Suggested Reading

Atug F, Castle EP, Burgess SV, Thomas R. Concomitant management of renal calculi and pelvi-ureteric junction obstruction with robotic laparoscopic surgery. BJU Int. 2005;96(9):1365–8.

Avlan D, Gündoğdu G, Delibaş A, Nayci A. Pyeloureterostomy in the management of the lower pole pelvi-ureteric junction obstruction in incomplete duplicated systems. Urology. 2010;76(6):1468–71.

Gonzalez F, Canning DA, Hyun G, Casale P. Lower pole pelvi-ureteric junction obstruction in duplicated collecting systems. BJU Int. 2006;97(1):161–5.

Goyal NK, Goel A, Yadav R. Conservative management of pelvi-ureteric junction obstruction (PUJO): is it appropriate and if so what duration of follow-up is needed? BJU Int. 2012;110(1):E1.

Groenen PM, Vanderlinden G, Devriendt K, Fryns JP, Van de Ven WJ. Rearrangement of the human CDC5L gene by a t(6;19)(p21;q13.1) in a patient with multicystic renal dysplasia. Genomics. 1998;49(2):218–29.

Manouvrier-Hanu S, Devisme L, Farre I, Hue V, Storme L, Kacet N, Boute-Benejean O, Farriaux JP. Pulmonary hypertension of the newborn and urogenital anomalies in two male siblings: a new family with misalignment of pulmonary vessels. Genet Couns. 1996;7(4):249–55.

S. S. Goonewardene et al., *Basic Urological Management*,
https://doi.org/10.1007/978-3-319-98720-0_70

Tasca A, Barulli M, Artibani W, Passerini G, Bui F, Cagnato P, Macri C. Role of the diuresis renogram in the study of the pelviureteric junction. Eur Urol. 1985;11(6):374–7.

Wah TM, Weston MJ, Irving HC. Lower moiety pelvic-ureteric junction obstruction (PUJO) of the duplex kidney presenting with pyonephrosis in adults. Br J Radiol. 2003;76(912):909–12.

Ward HC, Brereton RJ. Pelviureteric junction obstruction and recurrent abdominal pain in childhood. Br J Surg. 1989;76(8):818–9.

Management of PUJO

71

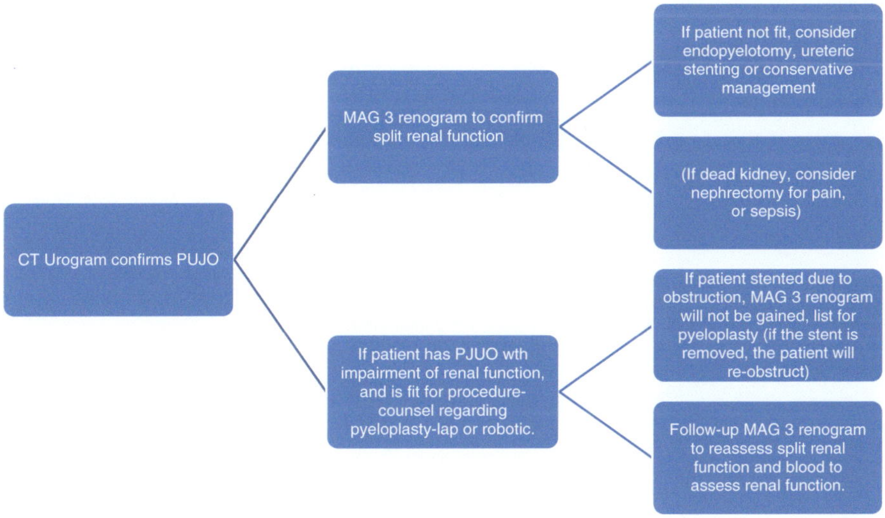

Suggested Reading

Atug F, Castle EP, Burgess SV, Thomas R. Concomitant management of renal calculi and pelvi-ureteric junction obstruction with robotic laparoscopic surgery. BJU Int. 2005;96(9):1365–8.

Avlan D, Gündoğdu G, Delibaş A, Nayci A. Pyeloureterostomy in the management of the lower pole pelvi-ureteric junction obstruction in incomplete duplicated systems. Urology. 2010;76(6):1468–71.

Gonzalez F, Canning DA, Hyun G, Casale P. Lower pole pelvi-ureteric junction obstruction in duplicated collecting systems. BJU Int. 2006;97(1):161–5.

Goyal NK, Goel A, Yadav R. Conservative management of pelvi-ureteric junction obstruction (PUJO): is it appropriate and if so what duration of follow-up is needed? BJU Int. 2012;110(1):E1.

S. S. Goonewardene et al., *Basic Urological Management*,
https://doi.org/10.1007/978-3-319-98720-0_71

Groenen PM, Vanderlinden G, Devriendt K, Fryns JP, Van de Ven WJ. Rearrangement of the human CDC5L gene by a t(6,19)(p21;q13.1) in a patient with multicystic renal dysplasia. Genomics. 1998;49(2):218–29.

Manouvrier-Hanu S, Devisme L, Farre I, Hue V, Storme L, Kacet N, Boute-Benejean O, Farriaux JP. Pulmonary hypertension of the newborn and urogenital anomalies in two male siblings: a new family with misalignment of pulmonary vessels. Genet Couns. 1996;7(4):249–55.

Tasca A, Barulli M, Artibani W, Passerini G, Bui F, Cagnato P, Macri C. Role of the diuresis renogram in the study of the pelviureteric junction. Eur Urol. 1985;11(6):374–7.

Wah TM, Weston MJ, Irving HC. Lower moiety pelvic-ureteric junction obstruction (PUJO) of the duplex kidney presenting with pyonephrosis in adults. Br J Radiol. 2003;76(912):909–12.

Ward HC, Brereton RJ. Pelviureteric junction obstruction and recurrent abdominal pain in childhood. Br J Surg. 1989;76(8):818–9.

Hydronephrosis

72

Definition

- Dilation of the renal pelvis
- May also include the ureter (hydro-ureteronephrosis)
- Usually due to an obstructive or functional cause
- Can be uni or bilateral
- If severe, can impair renal function.
- Has a number of causes

Causes

- Unilateral: ureteric/bladder tumour, prosate cancer, stones, infection, stricture, external compression, retroperitoneal fibrosis (Woodward et al).
- Bilateral: retention, prostate cancer, extensive bladder tumour, stones, reflux via re-implanted ureters.
- Pregnancy-usually right sided over left.
- Congenital anomalies (Toka)

History

- Flank pain (Mergener et al).
- UTIS.
- Fevers and rigors, sepsis.
- Nausea and vomiting.
- LUTS, retention.
- Haematuria-history of cancers, stones.

S. S. Goonewardene et al., *Basic Urological Management*,
https://doi.org/10.1007/978-3-319-98720-0_72

Examination

- Abdomen: Tenderness in flanks, palpable mass in flanks (?renal tumour/clot colic), palpable bladder (retention).
- Scrotal examination-assess for penile cancer, external urethral meatus (no phimosis)
- DRE-Size of prostate, volume, consisitency (?BPH/ Prostate cancer)

Investigations

- If flank pain-plain CT KUB-if contrast is used, you will not see stones.
- Bloods-FBC, CRP, U+Es.
- Urine anaysis and urine culture.
- If septic-septic screen and ABG-lactate.
- Haematuria-haematuria investigations-CT IVU EGFR >30 and flexible cystoscopy.
- If pregnant, USS KUB or MRI.
- If prostate cancer-PSA. If < 15, MRI and trasnperineal biopsy, if psa> 15 for bone scan.
- If penile cancer suspected, MRI penis.

Outcome

- Catheterise patient and measure residual
- Monitor renal function-if dernaged and not improving despite catheterisation, consider ureteric stent or nephrostomies
- Treat the cause
- If bladder cancer and localised, do a CT chest to complete staging and list to resect tumour. Once resected, the obstruction is removed and hydronephrosis should resolve, if not, consider ureteric stenting and removal of stent at a later date-foloow diagnostic pathway
- If prostate cancer-and patient fit for surgery/radiotherapy which should relieve obstruction-keep patient catheterised.
- IF penile cancer-if patietn fit consider listing for glansecotmy if superficial, or partial/total penectomy
- If stones, an patient obstrcted-follow pathway for renal colic

Suggested Reading

Mergener K, et al. Dietl's crisis: a syndrome of episodic abdominal pain of urologic origin that may present to a gastroenterologist. Am J Gastroenterol. 1997;92(12):2289–91.

Toka HR, Toka O, Hariri A, Nguyen HT. Congenital anomalies of kidney and urinary tract. Semin Nephrol. 2010;30(4):374–86.

Woodward M, Frank D. Postnatal management of antenatal hydronephrosis. BJU Int. 2010;89(2):149–56.

73 Diagnosis of Hydronephrosis

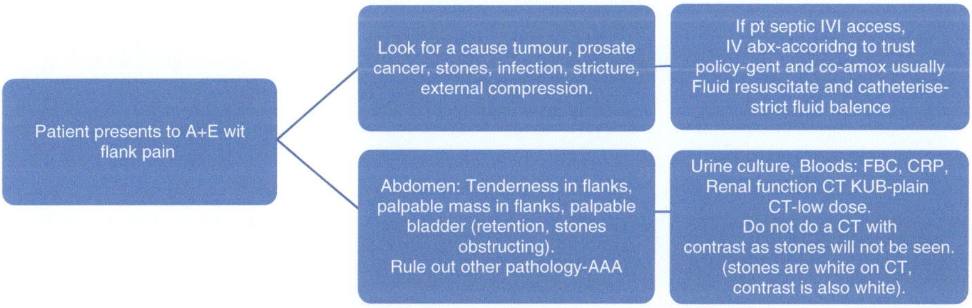

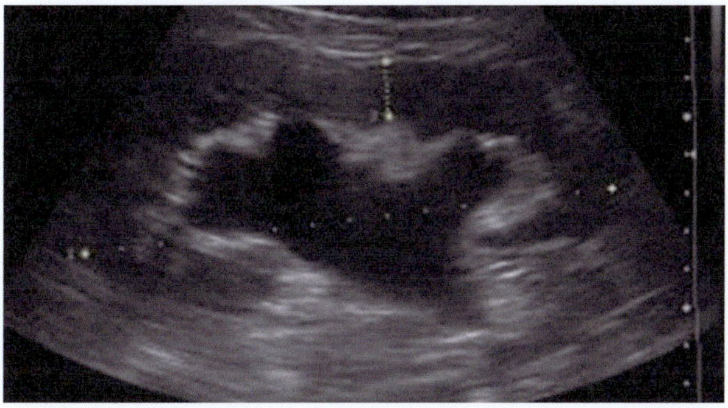

Fig. 73.1 Hydronephrosis on USS

S. S. Goonewardene et al., *Basic Urological Management*, https://doi.org/10.1007/978-3-319-98720-0_73

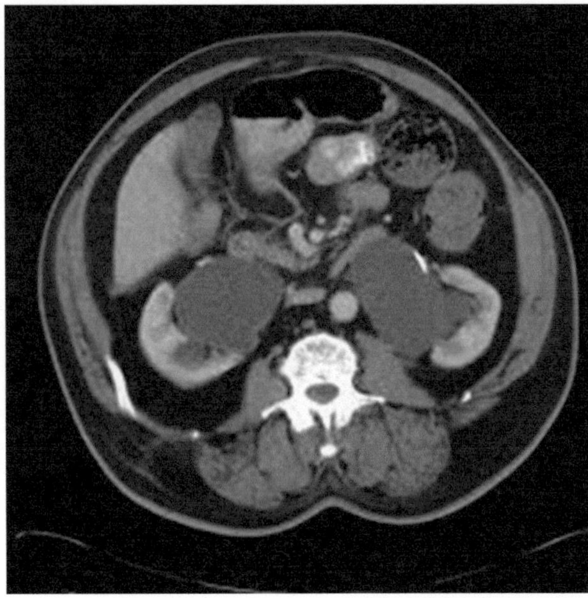

Fig. 73.2 Hydronephrosis on CT

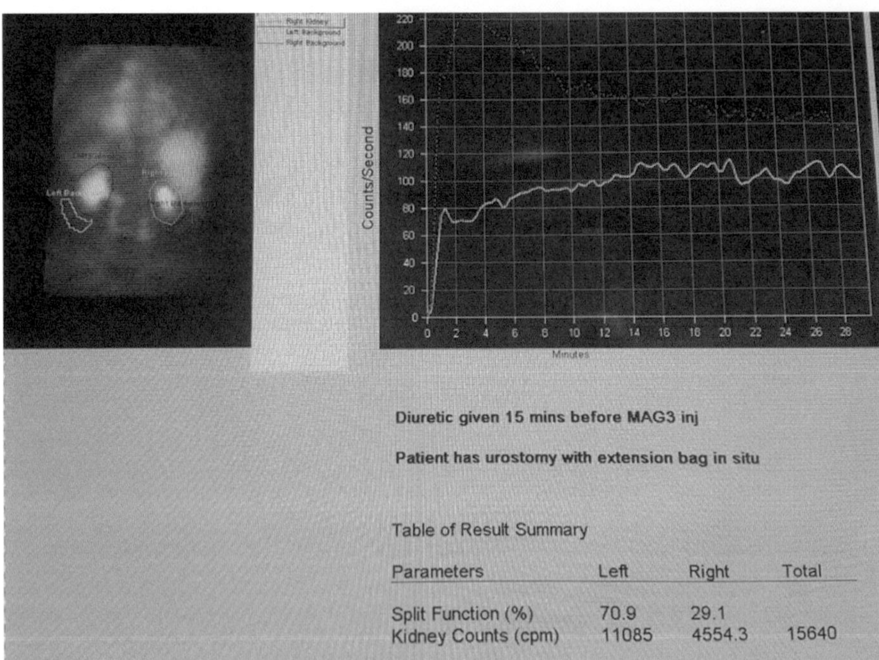

Fig. 73.3 MAG 3 demonstrating a right obstructed kidney, with uptake but poor excretion. Study conducted in a patient with ileostomy (urostomy)

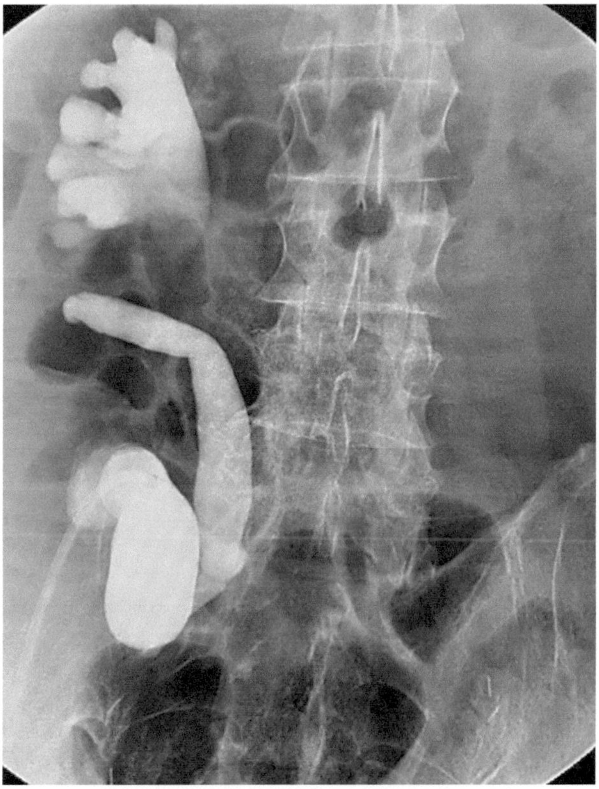

Fig. 73.4 An IVU conducted in same patient, demonstrating obstructive features—hydronephrosis and dilated calyces

Suggested Reading

Mergener K, et al. Dietl's crisis: a syndrome of episodic abdominal pain of urologic origin that may present to a gastroenterologist. Am J Gastroenterol. 1997;92(12):2289–91.

Toka HR, Toka O, Hariri A, Nguyen HT. Congenital anomalies of kidney and urinary tract. Semin Nephrol. 2010;30(4):374–86.

Woodward M, Frank D. Postnatal management of antenatal hydronephrosis. BJU Int. 2010;89(2):149–56.

Management of Hydronephrosis

74

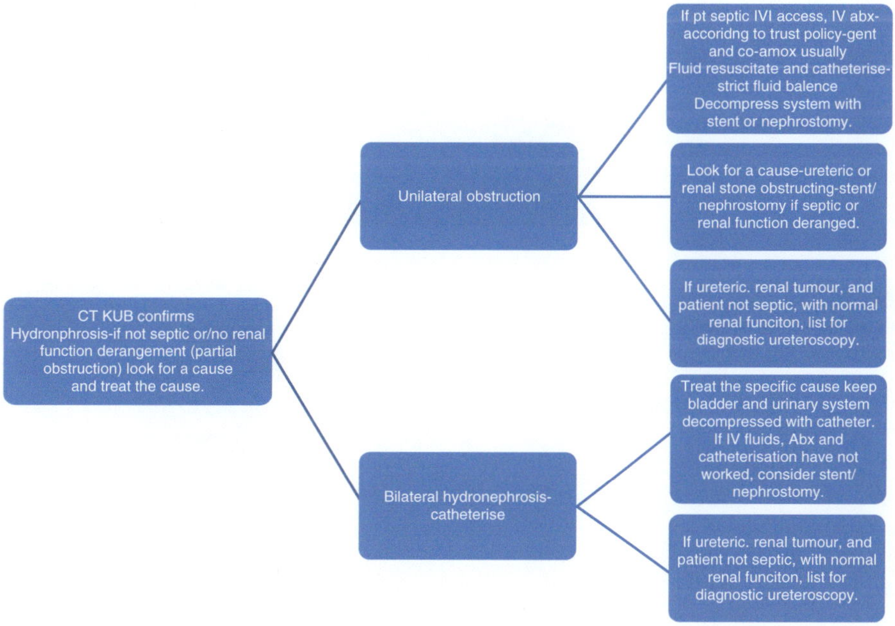

S. S. Goonewardene et al., *Basic Urological Management*,
https://doi.org/10.1007/978-3-319-98720-0_74

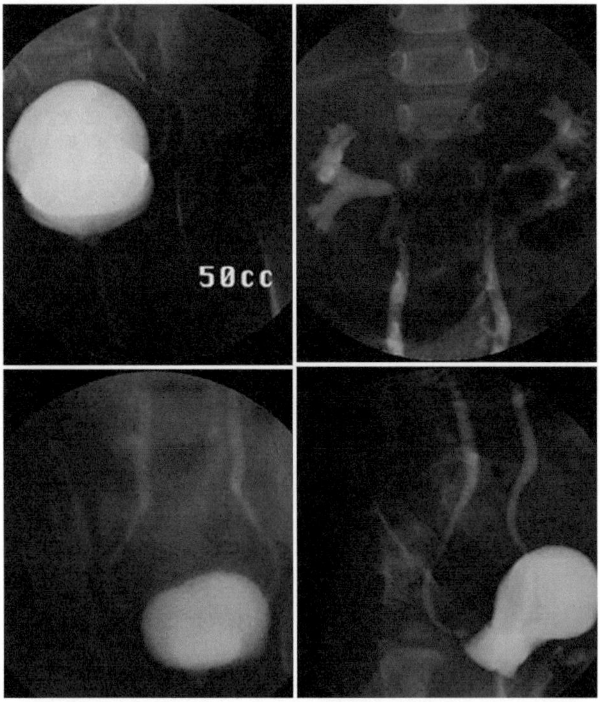

Fig. 74.1 An IVU demonstrating reflux

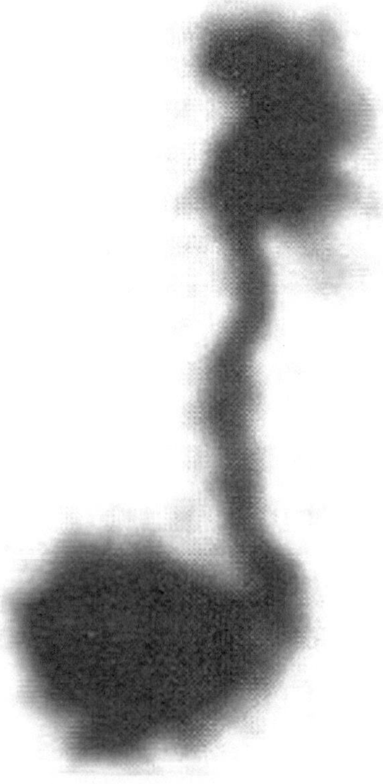

Fig. 74.2 An NM scan demonstrating severe reflux

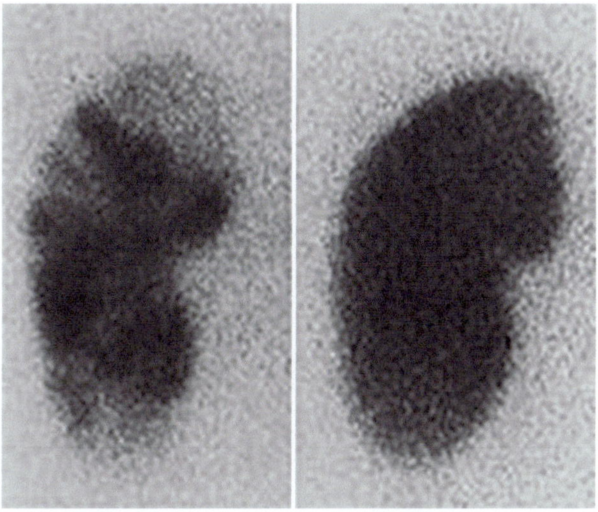

Fig. 74.3 Demonstrating a pyelonephritic kidney and normal kidney

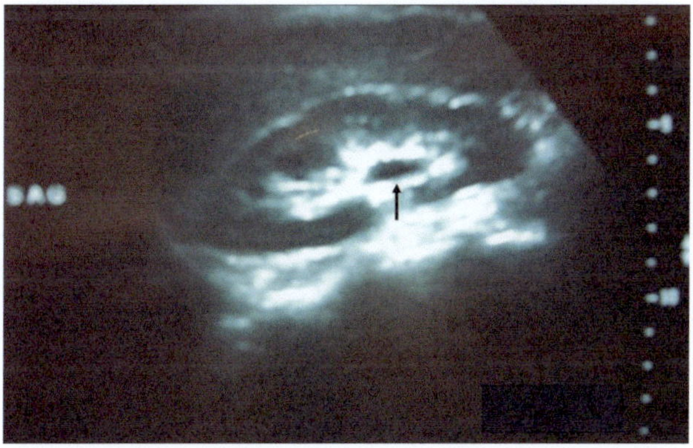

Fig. 74.4 USS demonstrating a lower pole hydronephrosis

Suggested Reading

Mergener K, et al. Dietl's crisis: a syndrome of episodic abdominal pain of urologic origin that may present to a gastroenterologist. Am J Gastroenterol. 1997;92(12):2289–91.

Toka HR, Toka O, Hariri A, Nguyen HT. Congenital anomalies of kidney and urinary tract. Semin Nephrol. 2010;30(4):374–86.

Woodward M, Frank D. Postnatal management of antenatal hydronephrosis. BJU Int. 2010;89(2):149–56.

75 Renal Trauma

Definition

- Damage to the renal parenchyma, collecting system or vasculature.
- Most commonly the result of a direct blow to the paravertebral gutter/flank.
- Can also happen as a part of RTCs, eg fall onto a side, off a motor bike.
- Is usually managed conservatively, unless haemodynamically unstable.
- Is graded 1–5, as per AAST trauma grading.
- Up to grade 4 can usually be managed conservatively long as patient is haemodynamically stable and not passing haematuria.

Causes

- Blunt trauma, falling on the side, or a blow to the flank (tends to be managed conservatively, if haemodynamically stable) Kautza et al.
- Deceleration type injuries
- Penetrating trauma-stab wound or gunshot

S. S. Goonewardene et al., *Basic Urological Management*,
https://doi.org/10.1007/978-3-319-98720-0_75

History

- History of trauma, when, where, how did it occur?
- Pain in the flank?
- Haematura or retention present?
- Loss of conciousness/dizziness
- Collateral history-allergies, past medical history, events leading up to trauma, last meal time.

Examination

- ATLS approach-ABCDE
- Abdomen: Tenderness in flanks, palpable mass in flanks (haematoma, expansile pulsatile mass-bleeding kidney), brusiing overflanks, palpable bladder (retention), penetraing wounds.
- Scrotal examination-blood at the external urethral meatus, intact scrotum?
- DRE.

Investigations

- Simultaneous assessment and management.
- ABCDE approach, observations.
- IV acess, bloods FBS, U+Es, LFTs, clotting and G+S.
- Catheterise.
- Trauma CT-keep patient in spinal immobilitation-request CT Urogram if renal function normal-triple phast CT, looking at vasculature and excretory phase.

Outcome

- Grades 1–4 managed conservatively wityh bedrest, IV acess and antibiotics.
- Keep patient catheterised to monitor urine output.
- Follow the patient up in outpatients in 6 weeks, advise the GP to monitor BP. (McCombie et al)
- Grade 5-shattered kidney, keep patient NBM, if haemodynamically unstable list for trauma nephrectomy. Contact vascular surgery, as part of this procedure involves clamping the aorta.
- If going to theatre, Crossmatch 4 units blood, FFP and platelets.
- An on table IVP would be conducted and vascular control would be obtained prior to trauma nephrectomy. (McClung et al, Yeung et al)

Suggested Reading

Kautza B, Zuckerbraun B, Peitzman AB. Management of blunt renal injury: what is new? Eur J Trauma Emerg Surg. 2015;41(3):251–8.

McClung CD, Hotaling JM, Wang J, Wessells H, Voelzke BB. Contemporary trends in the immediate surgical management of renal trauma using a national database. J Trauma Acute Care Surg. 2013;75(4):602–6.

McCombie SP, Thyer I, Corcoran NM, Rowling C, Dyer J, Le Roux A, Kuan M, Wallace DM, Hayne D. The conservative management of renal trauma: a literature review and practical clinical guideline from Australia and New Zealand. BJU Int. 2014;114(Suppl 1):13–21.

Yeung LL, Brandes SB. Contemporary management of renal trauma: differences between urologists and trauma surgeons. J Trauma Acute Care Surg. 2012;72(1):68–75; discussion 75–7.

76 Grading of Renal Trauma

Grade 1
- Contusion
- Subcapsular perirenal haematoma

Grade 2
- Superficial laceration <1 cm depth

Grade 3
- Laceration >1 cm

Grade 4
- Laceration extends to renal pelvis or urinary extravasation
- Renal artery or vein with contained haemorrhage
- Segmental infarctions without associated lacerations
- Expanding subcapsular haematomas

Grade 5
- Shattered kidney
- Avulsion of renal hilum: devascularisation of a kidney due to hilar injury
- Ureteropelvic avulsions
- Complete laceration or thrombus of the main renal artery or vein

S. S. Goonewardene et al., *Basic Urological Management*,
https://doi.org/10.1007/978-3-319-98720-0_76

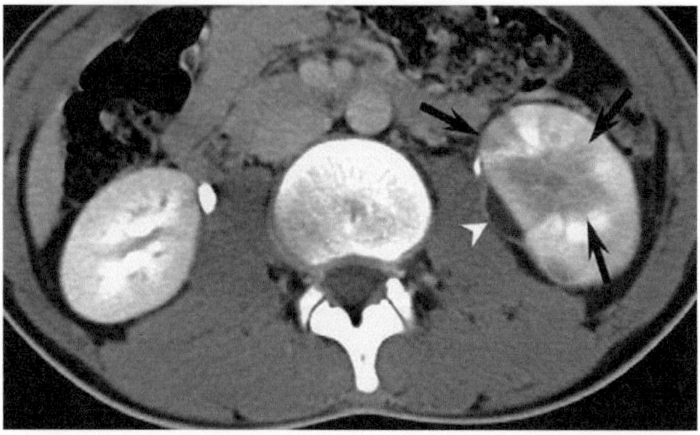

Fig. 76.1 Grade 1 renal trauma on CT

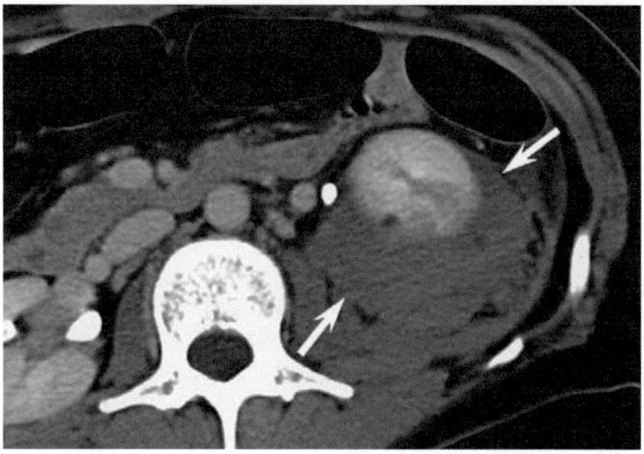

Fig. 76.2 Grade 2 renal trauma on CT

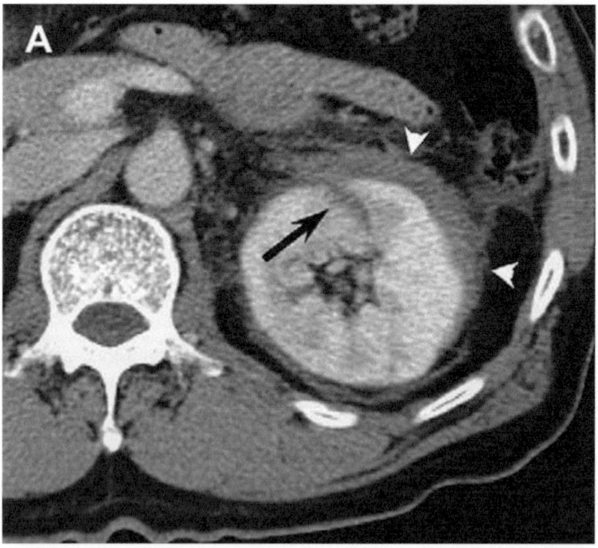

Fig. 76.3 Grade 3 renal trauma on CT

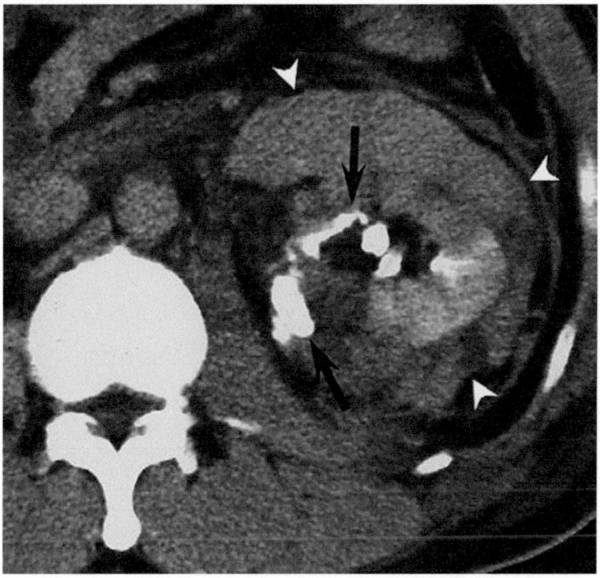

Fig. 76.4 Grade 4 renal trauma on CT

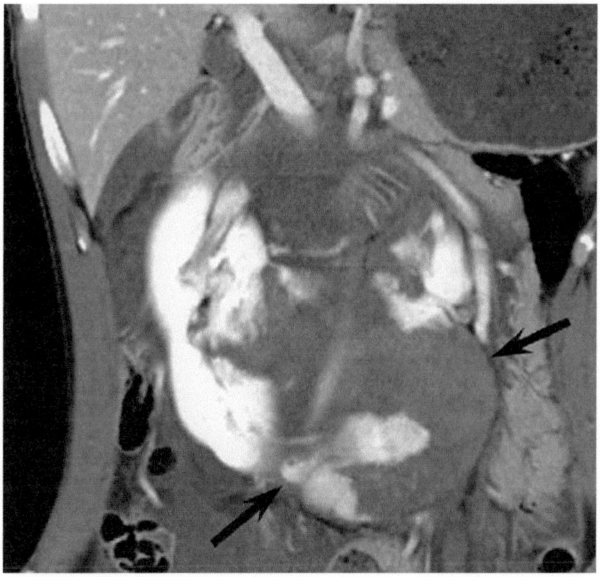

Fig. 76.5 Grade 5 renal trauma on CT

Suggested Reading

Croce MA, Fabian TC, Kudsk KA, Baum SL, Payne LW, Mangiante EC, Britt LG. AAST organ injury scale: correlation of CT-graded liver injuries and operative findings. J Trauma. 1991;31(6):806–12.

77 Diagnostic Pathway for Renal Trauma

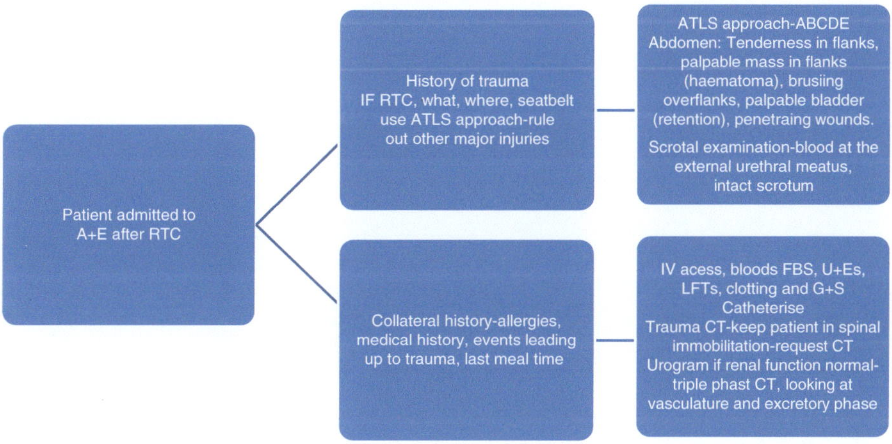

Suggested Reading

Kautza B, Zuckerbraun B, Peitzman AB. Management of blunt renal injury: what is new? Eur J Trauma Emerg Surg. 2015;41(3):251–8.

McClung CD, Hotaling JM, Wang J, Wessells H, Voelzke BB. Contemporary trends in the immediate surgical management of renal trauma using a national database. J Trauma Acute Care Surg. 2013;75(4):602–6.

McCombie SP, Thyer I, Corcoran NM, Rowling C, Dyer J, Le Roux A, Kuan M, Wallace DM, Hayne D. The conservative management of renal trauma: a literature review and practical clinical guideline from Australia and New Zealand. BJU Int. 2014;114(Suppl 1):13–21.

Yeung LL, Brandes SB. Contemporary management of renal trauma: differences between urologists and trauma surgeons. J Trauma Acute Care Surg. 2012;72(1):68–75. discussion 75–7.

S. S. Goonewardene et al., *Basic Urological Management*,
https://doi.org/10.1007/978-3-319-98720-0_77

Management Pathway for Renal Trauma

78

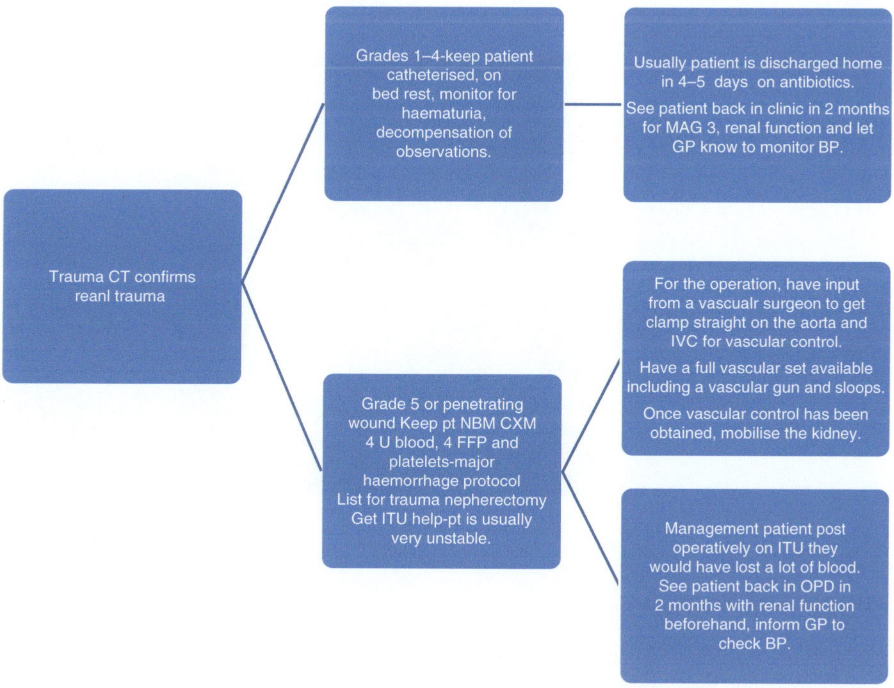

S. S. Goonewardene et al., *Basic Urological Management*,
https://doi.org/10.1007/978-3-319-98720-0_78

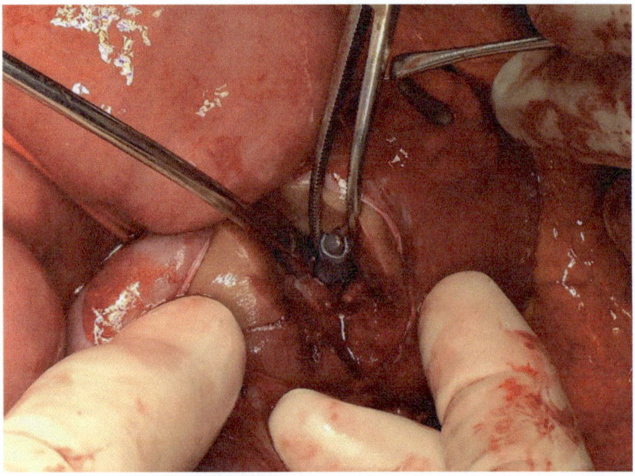

Fig. 78.1 Surgical management of renal trauma

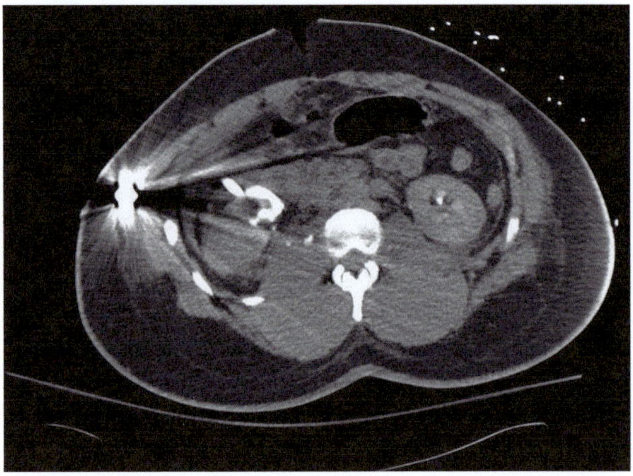

Fig. 78.2 Gunshot to the abdomen

Suggested Reading

Kautza B, Zuckerbraun B, Peitzman AB. Management of blunt renal injury: what is new? Eur J Trauma Emerg Surg. 2015;41(3):251–8.

McClung CD, Hotaling JM, Wang J, Wessells H, Voelzke BB. Contemporary trends in the immediate surgical management of renal trauma using a national database. J Trauma Acute Care Surg. 2013;75(4):602–6.

McCombie SP, Thyer I, Corcoran NM, Rowling C, Dyer J, Le Roux A, Kuan M, Wallace DM, Hayne D. The conservative management of renal trauma: a literature review and practical clinical guideline from Australia and New Zealand. BJU Int. 2014;114(Suppl 1):13–21.

Yeung LL, Brandes SB. Contemporary management of renal trauma: differences between urologists and trauma surgeons. J Trauma Acute Care Surg. 2012;72(1):68–75. discussion 75–7.

Ureteric Trauma

79

Definition

- Damage to the ureter, which may be partial or total.
- Commonly caused by ureteroscopy, colorectal surgery or gysecological or vascular surgery (Burks et al).
- Management depends on whether injury is total or partial, and position on the ureter (proximal, mid or distal).
- Immediate repair is ideal, but Injuries may be picked up some time after the surgery.
- Injury is graded 1–5 (Allen et al).

Causes

- Ureteroscopy-with a difficult ureter expecially with poor vision or a rought insertion of an access sheath, it is very easy to go through a ureter and into the abdomen-don't push a ureteroscope if vision is poor (Burks et al). (Watterson et al).
- Colorectal surgery, if the ureter is not properly identified, especially on the left, or not stented beforehand, it can be easy to damage, especially during a dififcult dissecion on the left side.
- Gynaecological surgery-during an abdominal hysterectomy.
- Penetrating trauma-gunshot, or knife (Bruno et al).

S. S. Goonewardene et al., *Basic Urological Management*,
https://doi.org/10.1007/978-3-319-98720-0_79

History

- Review the notes-if surgery beforehand, was it a difficult procedure, was the ureter identified, isolated and protected?
- Was the ureter pre-stented and easily identifiable as a result?
- Time since surgery or trauma-less than 24 hours or extending into weeks?
- If so nephrostomise and book for reconstruction in 2 months
- Patient symptoms: pain in the flank, haematuria, fevers/ rigors
- Collateral history-allergies, medical history, events leading up to trauma, last meal time.

Examination

- ATLS approach-ABCDE.
- Is the patient septic?
- Observations,-temperature, heart rate, RR.
- Abdomen: Tenderness in flanks, palpable mass in flanks (renal, urinoma, abcess), palpable bladder (retention), penetraing wounds/ surgical wounds.

Investigations

- Simultaneous assessment and management.
- ABCDE approach, note observations.
- IV acess, bloods FBS, U+Es, LFTs, clotting and G+S.
- Catheterise.
- If post surgery, CT urogram, to assess position (upper, mid, lower third) and extent of trauma to ureter (haematoma, <50% diameter, >50% diameter, total injury).

Outcome

- Ideal assessment is done at time of injury-rigid cystoscopy, retrogrades +/–stent and immediate repair (uretero-ureterostomy, transuretero-ureterostomy, psoas hitch or boari flap).
- if Haematoma (conservative management +/–stent), < 50% use ureteric stent.
- If > 50% may require repair-ureteroureterostomy / pelvicalycostomy (upper third injury), transureterourterostomy (mid third ureter), psoas hitch or boari flap (lower third).
- If detected after surgery, drain kidney via nephrostomy and reconstruct in 2 months.

Suggested Reading

Burks FN, Santucci RA. Management of iatrogenic ureteral injury. Ther Adv Urol. 2014;6(3):115–24.

Morey AF, Brandes S, Dugi DD III, Armstrong JH, Breyer BN, Broghammer JA, Erickson BA, Holzbeierlein J, Hudak SJ, Mirvis S, Pruitt JH, Reston JT, Santucci RA, Smith TG III, Wessells H. Urotrauma: AUA guideline. J Urol. 2014;192(2):327–35.

Pereira BMT, Ogilvie MP, Gomez-Rodriguez JC, Ryan ML, Peña D, Marttos AC, Pizano LR, McKenney MG. A review of ureteral injuries after external trauma. Scand J Trauma Resusc Emerg Med. 2010;18:6.

Watterson JD, Mahoney JE, Futter NG, Gaffield J. Iatrogenic ureteric injuries: approaches to etiology and management. Can J Surg. 1998;41(5):379–82.

Ureteric Injury Severity Scale

80

Grade 1
- Contusion
- Haematoma
- With or without devascularisation

Grade 2
- <50% transection of ureter

Grade 3
- >50% transection of ureter

Grade 4
- Complete transection
- < 2cm devascularisation

Grade 5
- Avulsion with > 2 cm devascularisation

S. S. Goonewardene et al., *Basic Urological Management*,
https://doi.org/10.1007/978-3-319-98720-0_80

Suggested Reading

Morey AF, Steve B, Dugi DD III, Armstrong JH, Breyer BN, Broghammer JA, Erickson BA, Holzbeierlein J, Hudak SJ, Mirvis S, Pruitt JH, Reston JT, Santucci RA, Smith TG III, Wessells H. Urotrauma: AUA guideline. J Urol. 2014;192(2):327–35.

81 Diagnostic Pathway for Ureteric Trauma

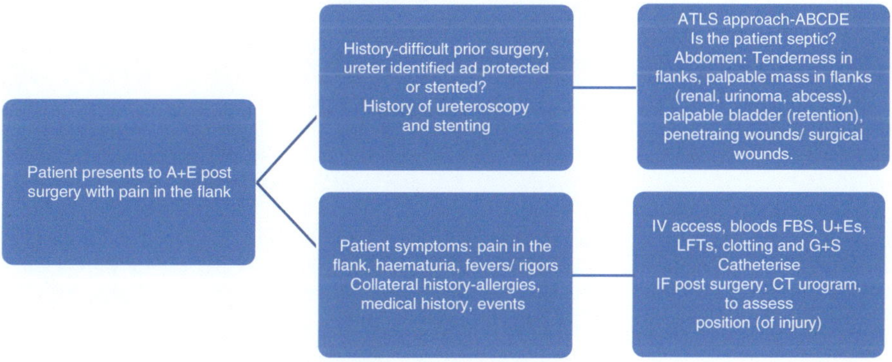

S. S. Goonewardene et al., *Basic Urological Management*,
https://doi.org/10.1007/978-3-319-98720-0_81

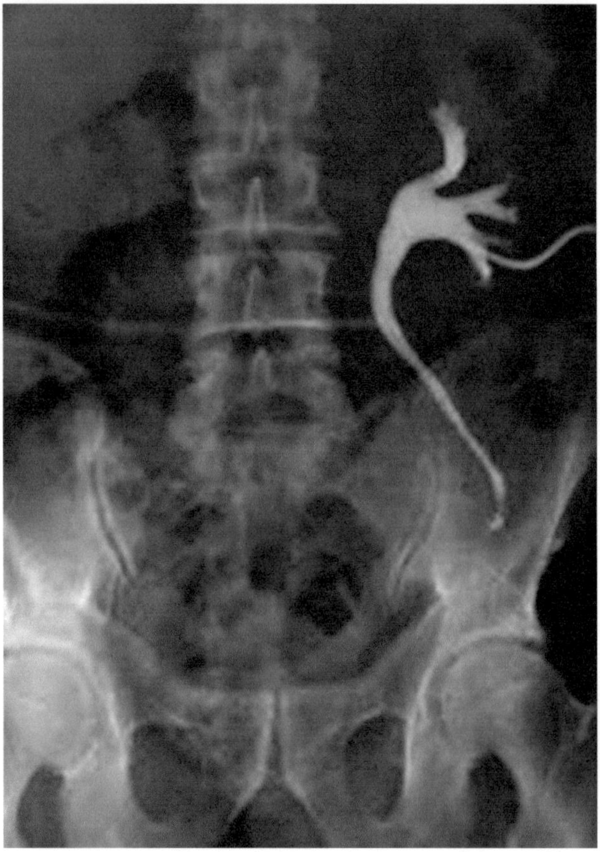

Fig. 81.1 IVU through a nephrostogram demonstrating ureteric injury (the contrast is not draining down throught the ureter to the bladder)

Suggested Reading

Burks FN, Santucci RA. Management of iatrogenic ureteral injury. Ther Adv Urol. 2014;6(3):115–24.

Morey AF, Steve B, Dugi DD III, Armstrong JH, Breyer BN, Broghammer JA, Erickson BA, Holzbeierlein J, Hudak SJ, Mirvis S, Pruitt JH, Reston JT, Santucci RA, Smith TG III, Wessells H. Urotrauma: AUA guideline. J Urol. 2014;192(2):327–35.

Pereira BMT, Ogilvie MP, Gomez-Rodriguez JC, Ryan ML, Peña D, Marttos AC, Pizano LR, McKenney MG. A review of ureteral injuries after external trauma. Scand J Trauma Resusc Emerg Med. 2010;18:6.

Watterson JD, Mahoney JE, Futter NG, Gaffield J. Iatrogenic ureteric injuries: approaches to etiology and management. Can J Surg. 1998;41(5):379–82.

Management of Ureteric Injury

82

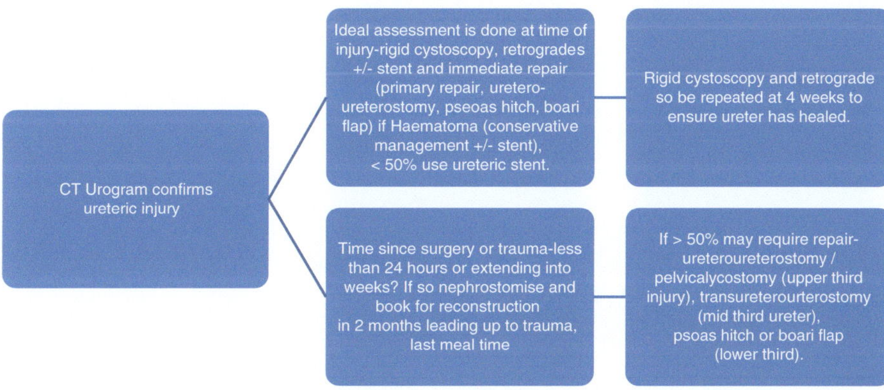

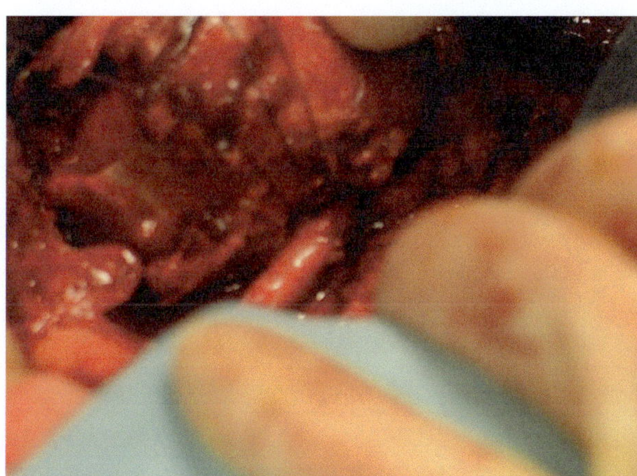

Fig. 82.1 Primary repair of a ureter

S. S. Goonewardene et al., *Basic Urological Management*,
https://doi.org/10.1007/978-3-319-98720-0_82

Suggested Reading

Burks FN, Santucci RA. Management of iatrogenic ureteral injury. Ther Adv Urol. 2014;6(3):115–24.

Morey AF, Brandes S, Dugi DD III, Armstrong JH, Breyer BN, Broghammer JA, Erickson BA, Holzbeierlein J, Hudak SJ, Mirvis S, Pruitt JH, Reston JT, Santucci RA, Smith TG III, Wessells H. Urotrauma: AUA guideline. J Urol. 2014;192(2):327–35.

Pereira BMT, Ogilvie MP, Gomez-Rodriguez JC, Ryan ML, Peña D, Marttos AC, Pizano LR, McKenney MG. A review of ureteral injuries after external trauma. Scand J Trauma Resusc Emerg Med. 2010;18:6.

Watterson JD, Mahoney JE, Futter NG, Gaffield J. Iatrogenic ureteric injuries: approaches to etiology and management. Can J Surg. 1998;41(5):379–82.

Bladder Trauma

83

Definition

- Damage to the bladder.
- Commonly caused by resection of tumour or cystoscopy, blows to a full bladder, gynaecological surgery, wearing a seatbelt across a full bladder.
- Management depends on whether injury is extra or intraperitoneal
- It is graded 1-5 (Allen et al).
- Check for associated rectal injury (Pereira et al).

Causes

- Transurethral resection of bladder tumour-some tumours are extensive and it is difficult to determine where the bladder wall is, as a result, resection of bladder wall can occur. Tumours at the done or anterior wall are more liable to have an intraperitoneal perforation.
- Cystoscopy or cystoscopy and biopsy-in elderly women, it is easy to pass a cystscope through a thin bladder wall.
- Gynaecological surgery-during an abdominal hysterectomy or c-section, it can be difficult to see the plane between the bladder and uterus-as a result, bladder trauma can occur.
- Penetrating trauma to the lower abdomen-gunshot, or knife (Uwais et al).
- Pelvic fractures.
- Blunt trauma to the lower abdomen (Kong et al).

S. S. Goonewardene et al., *Basic Urological Management*,
https://doi.org/10.1007/978-3-319-98720-0_83

History

- Review the notes-what were the events leading up to bladder trauma?
- Was it an RTC, was the patient restrained? Is there suprapubic pain, retention, or visible haematuria.
- If bladder injury during surgery, was the bladder identified, or was it a difficult procedure.
- Time since surgery or trauma-very often, especially if an extraperitoneal injury, patients present late.
- Collateral history-allergies, medical history, events leading up to trauma, last meal time, full bladder at time of incident.

Examination

- ATLS approach-ABCDE
- Is the patient septic?
- Abdomen: Tenderness in flanks, palpable mass in flanks (renal, urinoma, abcess), palpable bladder (retention), penetraing wounds/ surgical wounds.

Investigations

- Simultaneous assessment and management.
- ABCDE approach, obsrevations.
- IV acess, bloods FBS, U+Es, LFTs, clotting and G+S.
- Catheterise.
- A retrograde cystogram to assess extent of injury-whether extra or intraperitoneal (needs at least 400 mls of contrast in the bladder to demonstrate injury).
- If no leak is demonstrated, it may just be bladder contusion.
- Exrta and Intra peritoneal leakages may be demosnstrated.
- if injury occurs on table, assess the extent and degree of severity of injury.

Outcome

- Ideal assessment is done at time of injury-immediate repair if patient has an open procedure.-mass closure of the bladder with absorbable interrupted sutures.
- If done during resection of tumour, do an on table cystogram, to assess whether extraperionteal or intraperitoneal.
- If extraperiteoneal, catheterise for two weeks and then do a pericatheter cystogram.
- If there is no leak, remove catheter.
- The indications for surgery with extraperitoneal rupture are clot retention, pelvic bone puncturing bladder wall, bladder not healing with extravasation ongoing, bladder neck injury, undergoing open surgery for other procedures.
- If intraperitoneal, patient requires lower midline laparotomy and formal closure of the bladder.
- If patient presents as an outpatient, conduct a retrograde cystogram immediately and keep the patient catheterised.

Suggested Reading

Kong JPL, Bultitude MF, Royce P, Gruen RL, Cato A, Corcoran NM. Lower urinary tract injuries following blunt trauma: a review of contemporary management. Rev Urol. 2011;13(3):119–30.

Morey AF, Brandes S, Dugi DD III, Armstrong JH, Breyer BN, Broghammer JA, Erickson BA, Holzbeierlein J, Hudak SJ, Mirvis S, Pruitt JH, Reston JT, Santucci RA, Smith TG III, Wessells H. Urotrauma: AUA guideline. J Urol. 2014;192(2):327–35.

Pereira BM, Reis LO, Calderan TR, de Campos CC, Fraga GP. Penetrating bladder trauma: a high risk factor for associated rectal injury. Adv Urol. 2014;2014:386280.

Zaid UB, Bayne DB, Harris CR, Alwaal A, McAninch JW, Breyer BN. Penetrating trauma to the ureter, bladder, and urethra. Curr Trauma Rep. 2015;1(2):119–24.

84 Injury Severity Scale, Bladder Trauma

Grade 1
- Contusion, intramural haematoma
- Partial thickness laceration

Grade 2
- Extraperitoneal bladder wall laceration <2cm

Grade 3
- Extraperitoneal laceration >2cm
- Intraperitoneal (<2cm) bladder wall laceration

Grade 4
- Intraperitoneal bladder wall laceration ≥2cm

Grade 5
- Intraperitoneal or extraperitoneal bladder wall laceration extending into the bladder neck or ureteral orifice (trigone)

Suggested Reading

Morey AF, Brandes S, Dugi DD III, Armstrong JH, Breyer BN, Broghammer JA, Erickson BA, Holzbeierlein J, Hudak SJ, Mirvis S, Pruitt JH, Reston JT, Santucci RA, Smith TG III, Wessells H. Urotrauma: AUA guideline. J Urol. 2014;192(2):327–35.

S. S. Goonewardene et al., *Basic Urological Management*,
https://doi.org/10.1007/978-3-319-98720-0_84

Diagnosis of Bladder Trauma

85

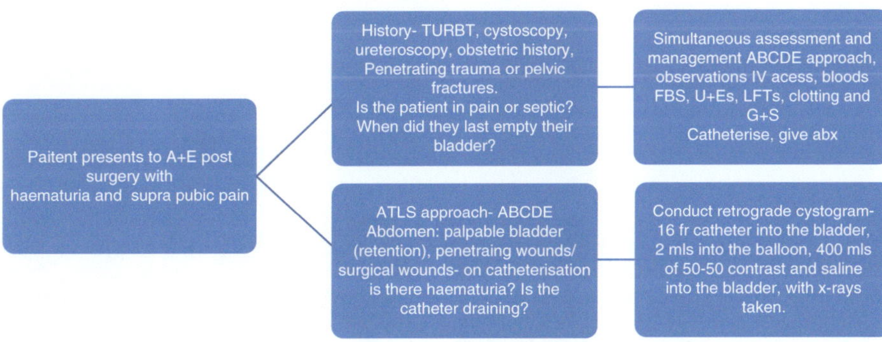

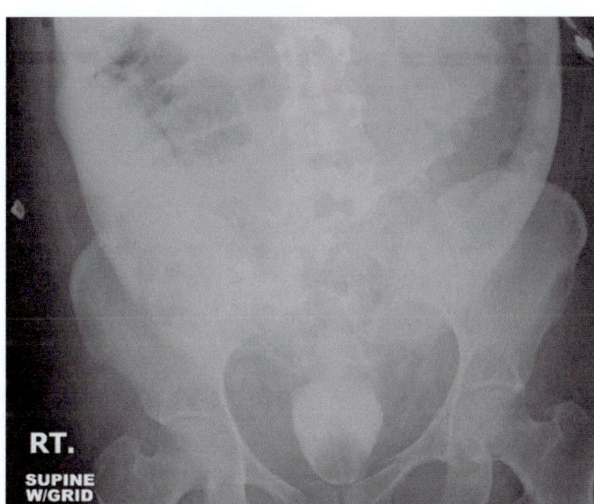

Fig. 85.1 Cystogram demonstrating intraperitoneal leakage

S. S. Goonewardene et al., *Basic Urological Management*,
https://doi.org/10.1007/978-3-319-98720-0_85

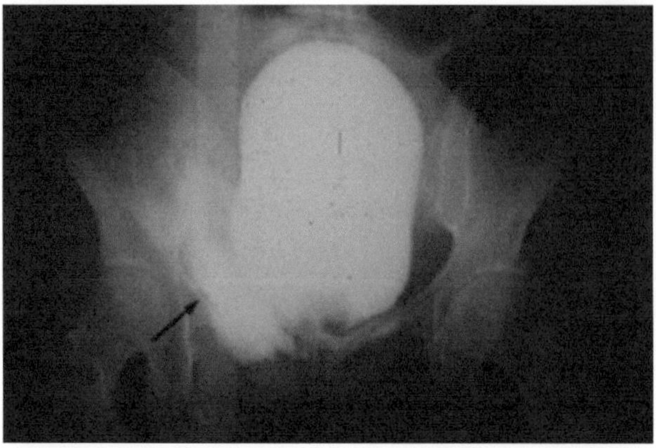

Fig. 85.2 Cystogram demonstrating extraperitoneal leakage

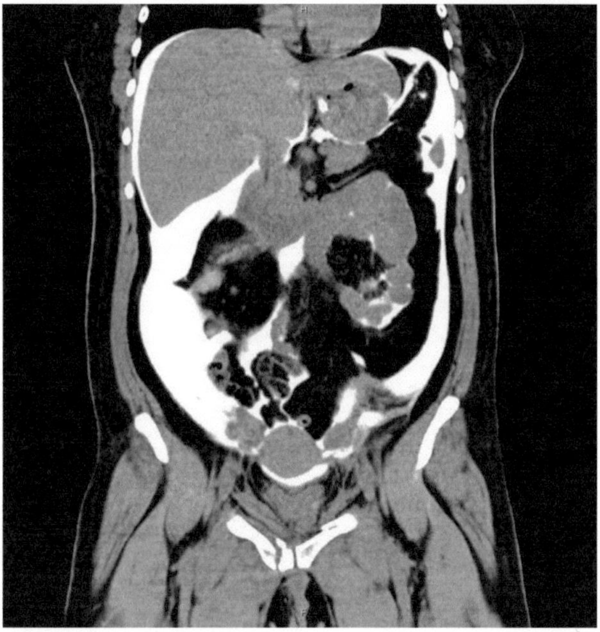

Fig. 85.3 CT demonstrating bladder trauma-leakage of contrast around abdomen (intraperitoneal leakage)

Suggested Reading

Kong JPL, Bultitude MF, Royce P, Gruen RL, Cato A, Corcoran NM. Lower urinary tract injuries following blunt trauma: a review of contemporary management. Rev Urol. 2011;13(3):119–30.

Morey AF, Steve B, Dugi DD III, Armstrong JH, Breyer BN, Broghammer JA, Erickson BA, Holzbeierlein J, Hudak SJ, Mirvis S, Pruitt JH, Reston JT, Santucci RA, Smith TG III, Wessells H. Urotrauma: AUA guideline. J Urol. 2014;192(2):327–35.

Pereira BM, Reis LO, Calderan TR, de Campos CC, Fraga GP. Penetrating bladder trauma: a high risk factor for associated rectal injury. Ther Adv Urol. 2014;2014:386280.

Zaid UB, Bayne DB, Harris CR, Alwaal A, McAninch JW, Breyer BN. Penetrating trauma to the ureter, bladder, and urethra. Curr Trauma Rep. 2015;1(2):119–24.

Management of Bladder Trauma

86

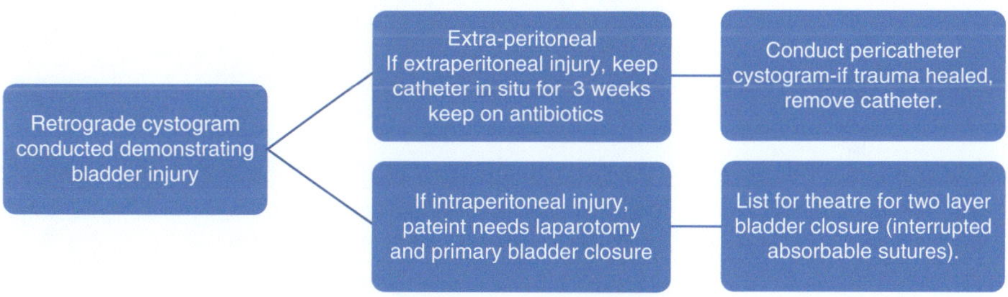

S. S. Goonewardene et al., *Basic Urological Management*,
https://doi.org/10.1007/978-3-319-98720-0_86

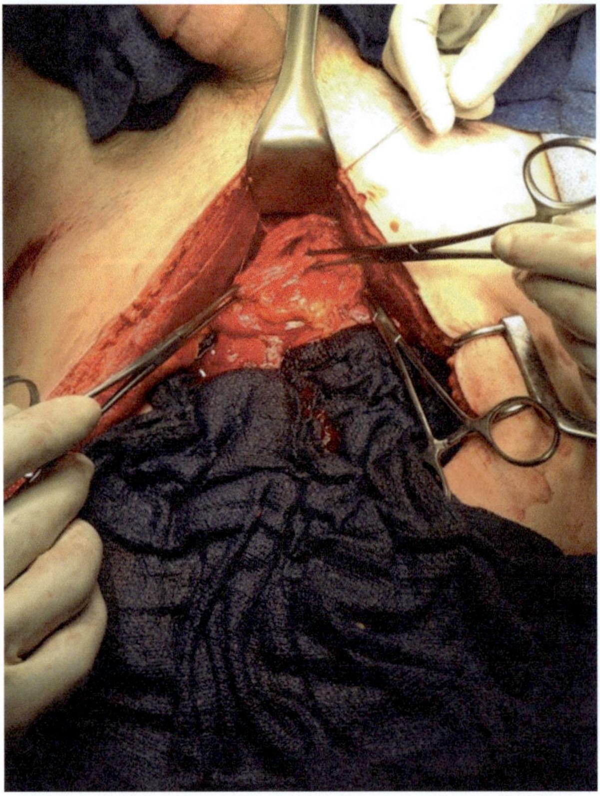

Fig. 86.1 Demonstrating repair of intraperitoneal bladder rupture-interrupted closure with absorbable sutures

Suggested Reading

Kong JPL, Bultitude MF, Royce P, Gruen RL, Cato A, Corcoran NM. Lower urinary tract injuries following blunt trauma: a review of contemporary management. Rev Urol. 2011;13(3):119–30.

Morey AF, Brandes S, Dugi DD III, Armstrong JH, Breyer BN, Broghammer JA, Erickson BA, Holzbeierlein J, Hudak SJ, Mirvis S, Pruitt JH, Reston JT, Santucci RA, Smith TG III, Wessells H. Urotrauma: AUA guideline. J Urol. 2014;192(2):327–35.

Pereira BM, Reis LO, Calderan TR, de Campos CC, Fraga GP. Penetrating bladder trauma: a high risk factor for associated rectal injury. Adv Urol. 2014;2014:386280.

Zaid UB, Bayne DB, Harris CR, Alwaal A, McAninch JW, Breyer BN. Penetrating trauma to the ureter, bladder, and urethra. Curr Trauma Rep. 2015;1(2):119–24.

Urethral Trauma

87

Definition

- Damage to the urethra which maybe partial or total.
- Can be anterior (saddle injury/ penile fracture) or posterior (pelvic fracture).
- Management depends on whether injury is total or partial.
- Urinary diversion with and SPC is required
- It is graded from 1–5 (Allen et al).

Causes

- Anterior-cycling injuries-straddle injuries or Penile fracture.
- Posterior-pelvic fracture.
- Blunt trauma.
- Penetraining trauma (Uwais et al).
- (McGready et al)

S. S. Goonewardene et al., *Basic Urological Management*,
https://doi.org/10.1007/978-3-319-98720-0_87

History

- Trauma-extent, degree, type.
- Patient symptoms:
  - SPC pain, retention, haematuria, fevers/ rigors, bruising on the perineum.
  - History of any foreign objects being passed into urethra.
- Collateral history-allergies, medical history, events leading up to trauma, last meal time.

Examination

- ATLS approach-ABCDE
- Is the patient septic?
- Abdomen:
  - Palpable bladder (retention)
  - Penetraing wounds/ surgical wounds
  - Bruising in the perineum
  - Blood at the meatus

Investigations

- Simultaneous assessment and management.
- ABCDE approach, observations.
- IV access, bloods FBS, U+Es, LFTs, clotting and G+S.
- Catheterise do not force the catheter, if unable to pass urethrally, place and SPC.
- Trauma CT.
- Urethrogram-30 degree oblique position bottom leg flexed at the hip and the knee.

Outcome

- If able to pass catheter-drain bladder and pericatheter urethogram in 2 weeks.
- If urethra is intact, twock.
- If strictures present, assess length for management-optical urethrtomy or primary reconstruction in 3 months.
- If unable to pass catheter-SPC to drain bladder or open cystostomy if pelvic haematoma.
- At a later date conduct voiding cysturethrography and twock if no strictures and no disruption of urethra.
- If urethra disrupted, keep catheterised and book for reconstrcution in 3 months at a specialist centre.

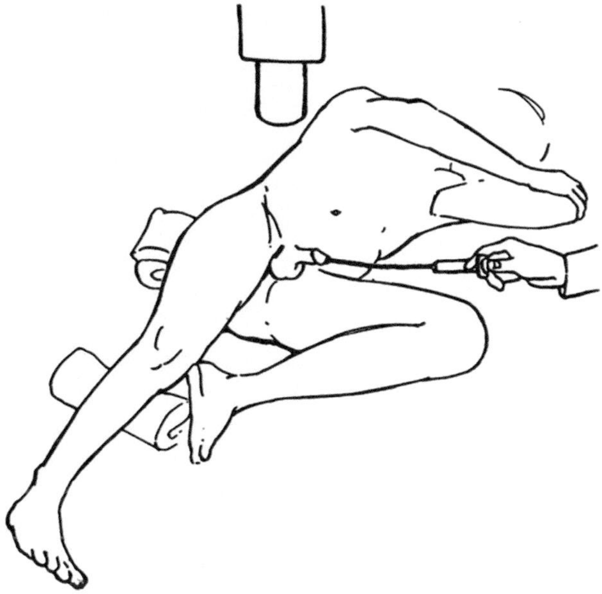

Fig. 87.1 Position of patient for urethrogram

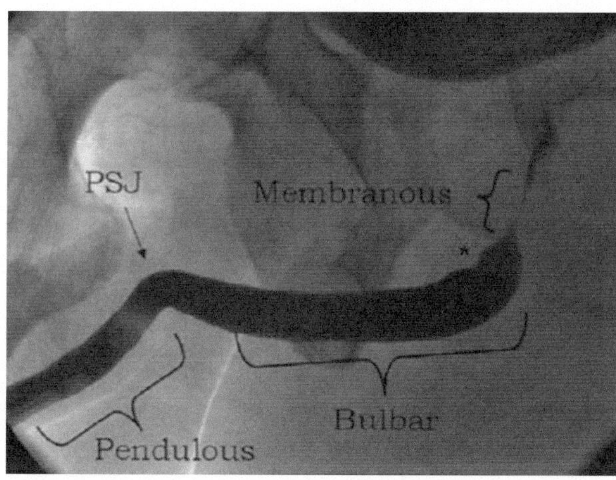

Fig. 87.2 Normal urethrogram

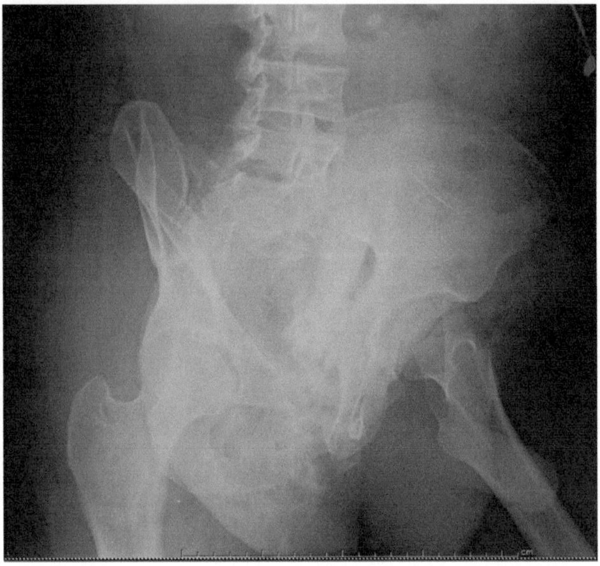

Fig. 87.3 Urethrogram demonstrating a posterior urethral injury

Suggested Reading

McGeady JB, Breyer BN. Current epidemiology of genitourinary trauma. Urol Clin North Am. 2013;40(3):323–33.

Morey AF, Brandes S, Dugi DD III, Armstrong JH, Breyer BN, Broghammer JA, Erickson BA, Holzbeierlein J, Hudak SJ, Mirvis S, Pruitt JH, Reston JT, Santucci RA, Smith TG III, Wessells H. Urotrauma: AUA guideline. J Urol. 2014;192(2):327–35.

Zaid UB, Bayne DB, Harris CR, Alwaal A, McAninch JW, Breyer BN. Penetrating trauma to the ureter, bladder, and urethra. Curr Trauma Rep. 2015;1(2):119–24.

88 Urethral Injury Severity Scoring

Grade 1

- Contusion
- Blood at urethral meatus; retrography normal

Grade 2

- Stretch injury
- Elongation of urethra without extravasation on urethrography

Grade 3

- Partial disruption
- Extravasation of urethrography contrast at injury site with visualization in the bladder

Grade 4

- Complete disruption
- Extravasation of urethrography contrast at injury site without visualization in the bladder
- <2cm of urethra separation

Grade 5

- Complete disruption
- Complete transaction with >2 cm urethral separation
- Extension into the prostate or vagina

S. S. Goonewardene et al., *Basic Urological Management*,
https://doi.org/10.1007/978-3-319-98720-0_88

Suggested Reading

Morey AF, Brandes S, Dugi DD III, Armstrong JH, Breyer BN, Broghammer JA, Erickson BA, Holzbeierlein J, Hudak SJ, Mirvis S, Pruitt JH, Reston JT, Santucci RA, Smith TG III, Wessells H. Urotrauma: AUA guideline. J Urol. 2014;192(2):327–35.

Diagnosis of Urethral Trauma

89

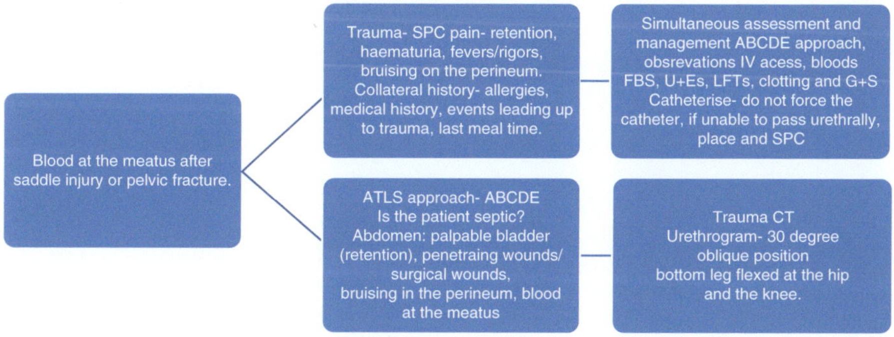

Suggested Reading

McGeady JB, Breyer BN. Current epidemiology of genitourinary trauma. Urol Clin North Am. 2013;40(3):323–33.

Morey AF, Brandes S, Dugi DD III, Armstrong JH, Breyer BN, Broghammer JA, Erickson BA, Holzbeierlein J, Hudak SJ, Mirvis S, Pruitt JH, Reston JT, Santucci RA, Smith TG III, Wessells H. Urotrauma: AUA guideline. J Urol. 2014;192(2):327–35.

Zaid UB, Bayne DB, Harris CR, Alwaal A, McAninch JW, Breyer BN. Penetrating trauma to the ureter, bladder, and urethra. Curr Trauma Rep. 2015;1(2):119–24.

S. S. Goonewardene et al., *Basic Urological Management*,
https://doi.org/10.1007/978-3-319-98720-0_89

90 Management Urethral Trauma

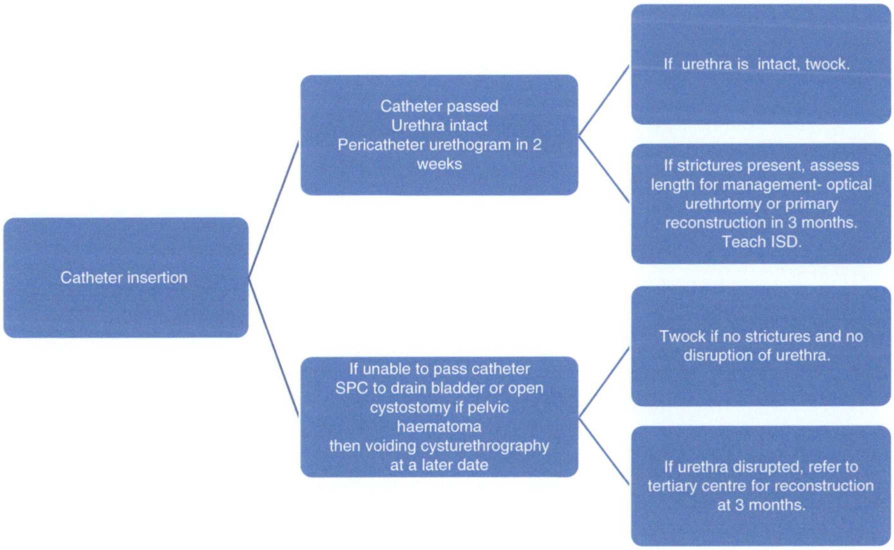

Suggested Reading

McGeady JB, Breyer BN. Current epidemiology of genitourinary trauma. Urol Clin North Am. 2013;40(3):323–33.

Morey AF, Steve B, Dugi DD III, Armstrong JH, Breyer BN, Broghammer JA, Erickson BA, Holzbeierlein J, Hudak SJ, Mirvis S, Pruitt JH, Reston JT, Santucci RA, Smith TG III, Wessells H. Urotrauma: AUA guideline. J Urol. 2014;192(2):327–35.

Zaid UB, Bayne DB, Harris CR, Alwaal A, McAninch JW, Breyer BN. Penetrating trauma to the ureter, bladder, and urethra. Curr Trauma Rep. 2015;1(2):119–24.

S. S. Goonewardene et al., *Basic Urological Management*,
https://doi.org/10.1007/978-3-319-98720-0_90

91 Testicular Trauma

Definition

- A blow to the testicle, which may cause rupture to the tunica albuginea
- The defining factor for surgical intervention, is whether the tunica albuginea is intact or not, and whether the skin is breached.
- Rule out other injuries.
- It it graded 1–5 (Allen et al).

Causes

- A blow to the testicle in sports.
- Blunt or penetrating trauma.
- A straddle injury to the scrotum.
- In a trauma patient, assess for testicular injury.

S. S. Goonewardene et al., *Basic Urological Management*,
https://doi.org/10.1007/978-3-319-98720-0_91

History

- A history of a blow to the testicles-time since the injury
- A history of trauma to the scrotal region.
- Associated skin lacerations, swelling or bruising to the scrotum.
- Events leading up to trauma, histroy of event, associated injuries, pelvic fractures, allergies, medications.

Examination

- ATLS approach.
- Primary survey.
- Review the abdomen: palpable bladder, masses/bruising in the flanks (renal trauma).
- Is there bloood at the external meatus? Rule out bladder and urethral trauma.
- Examine each hemiscrotum in turn, for swelling, pain, skin laceration, are the testes palpable and intact? (Naseer et al).

Investigation

- Bloods including FBC, U+Es, CRP, LFTs and clotting.
- If the skin is intact, USS the scrotum to determine if the tunica albuginea is intact or breached and to determine the blood supply to the testicle.
- USS with contrast enhancement also has a role in assessment of the testicle prior to exploration (Hedayati).
- If the skin is breached, the patient will need to go to theatre for exploration and closure.
- If the testicle is none viable, consent for prosthesis at a later date (Jacob et al).

Management

- Ultimately, if the tunica is not intact, surgical exploration will be needed.
- If the skin is closed, USS of scrotum, to determine this.
- If the skin of the scrotum is opened, or there is testicular rupture, formal exploration in theatre and closure will be required.
- Check tetanus status, and give a shot if indicated.

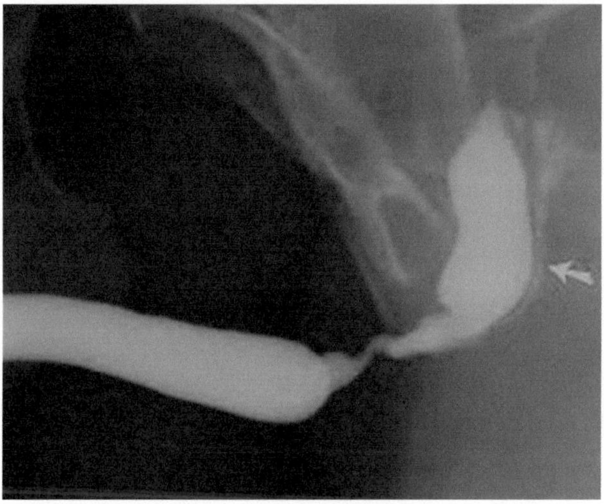

Fig. 91.1 Urogram demonstrating urethral trauma

Suggested Reading

Hedayati V, Sellars ME, Sharma DM, Sidhu PS. Contrast-enhanced ultrasound in testicular trauma: role in directing exploration, debridement and organ salvage. Br J Radiol. 2012;85(1011):e065–8.

Lucas JW, Lester KM, Chen A, Simhan J. Scrotal reconstruction and testicular prosthetics. Transl Androl Urol. 2017;6(4):710–21.

Morey AF, Brandes S, Dugi DD III, Armstrong JH, Breyer BN, Broghammer JA, Erickson BA, Holzbeierlein J, Hudak SJ, Mirvis S, Pruitt JH, Reston JT, Santucci RA, Smith TG III, Wessells H. Urotrauma: AUA guideline. J Urol. 2014;192(2):327–35.

Naseer A, King D, Lee H, Vale J. Testicular dislocation: the importance of scrotal examination in a trauma patient. Ann R Coll Surg Engl. 2012;94(2):e109–10.

Testicular Trauma Injury Scale

92

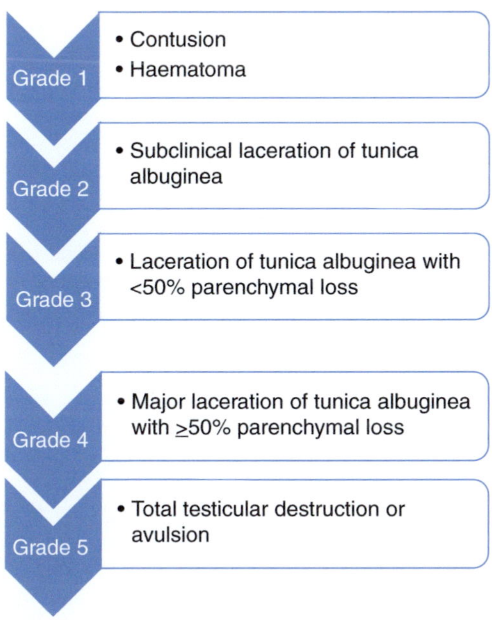

Suggested Reading

1. Morey AF, Brandes S, Dugi DD III, Armstrong JH, Breyer BN, Broghammer JA, Erickson BA, Holzbeierlein J, Hudak SJ, Mirvis S, Pruitt JH, Reston JT, Santucci RA, Smith TG III, Wessells H. Urotrauma: AUA guideline. J Urol. 2014;192(2):327–35.

S. S. Goonewardene et al., *Basic Urological Management*,
https://doi.org/10.1007/978-3-319-98720-0_92

Diagnosis of Testicular Trauma

93

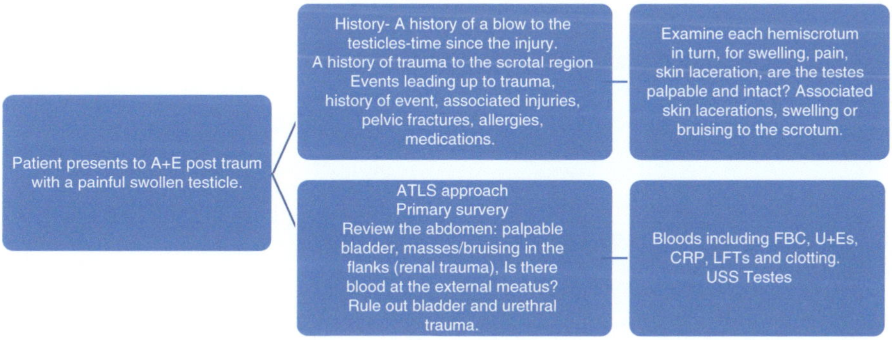

Suggested Reading

Hedayati V, Sellars ME, Sharma DM, Sidhu PS. Contrast-enhanced ultrasound in testicular trauma: role in directing exploration, debridement and organ salvage. Br J Radiol. 2012;85(1011):e065–8.

Lucas JW, Lester KM, Chen A, Simhan J. Scrotal reconstruction and testicular prosthetics. Transl Androl Urol. 2017;6(4):710–21.

Morey AF, Brandes S, Dugi DD III, Armstrong JH, Breyer BN, Broghammer JA, Erickson BA, Holzbeierlein J, Hudak SJ, Mirvis S, Pruitt JH, Reston JT, Santucci RA, Smith TG III, Wessells H. Urotrauma: AUA guideline. J Urol. 2014;192(2):327–35.

Naseer A, King D, Lee H, Vale J. Testicular dislocation: the importance of scrotal examination in a trauma patient. Ann R Coll Surg Engl. 2012;94(2):e109–10.

S. S. Goonewardene et al., *Basic Urological Management*,
https://doi.org/10.1007/978-3-319-98720-0_93

94 Management of Testicular Trauma

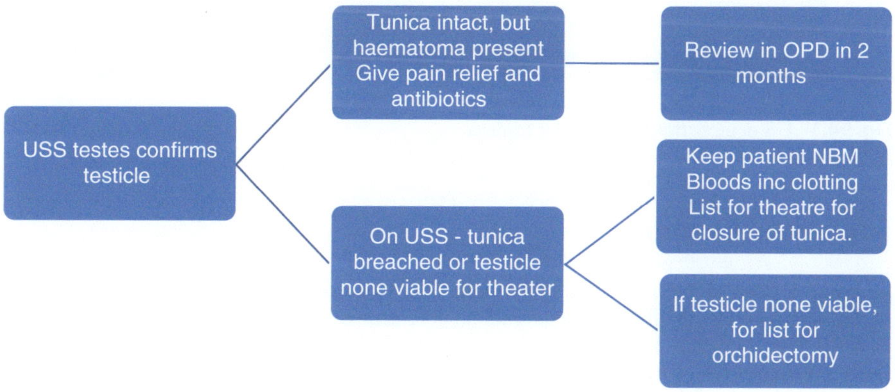

S. S. Goonewardene et al., *Basic Urological Management*,
https://doi.org/10.1007/978-3-319-98720-0_94

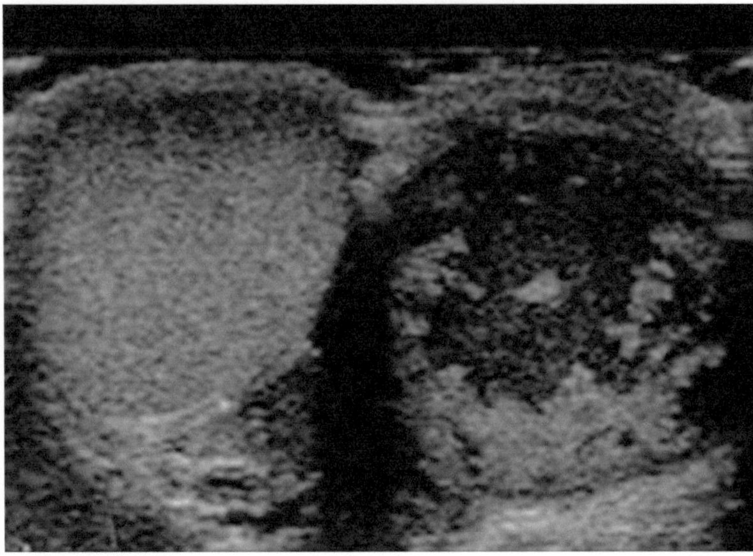

Fig. 94.1 US demonstrating testicular trauma

Suggested Reading

Hedayati V, Sellars ME, Sharma DM, Sidhu PS. Contrast-enhanced ultrasound in testicular trauma: role in directing exploration, debridement and organ salvage. Br J Radiol. 2012;85(1011):e065–8.

Lucas JW, Lester KM, Chen A, Simhan J. Scrotal reconstruction and testicular prosthetics. Transl Androl Urol. 2017;6(4):710–21.

Morey AF, Brandes S, Dugi DD III, Armstrong JH, Breyer BN, Broghammer JA, Erickson BA, Holzbeierlein J, Hudak SJ, Mirvis S, Pruitt JH, Reston JT, Santucci RA, Smith TG III, Wessells H. Urotrauma: AUA guideline. J Urol. 2014;192(2):327–35.

Naseer A, King D, Lee H, Vale J. Testicular dislocation: the importance of scrotal examination in a trauma patient. Ann R Coll Surg Engl. 2012;94(2):e109–10.

95 Overactive Bladder

Definition

- Bladder overactivity-urgency, with or without incontinence, frequency and nocturia.
- Symptoms can be irritative in nature.
- If diagnosed on urodynamics, with no evidence of cause, it is known as idiopathic detrusor overactivity.

Potential causes of symptoms-

- Bladder outfow obstruction-BPH, prostate cancer, prostatic stricture, prosatatitis.
- Infectious causes-UTIS, stones, cystitis.
- Neuropathic causes-Diabetes, lower motor neuron disease.
- Gynaecological: ovarian or uterine mass, preganancy.
- Caffeine or fluid intake, urethral diverticula or urethral caruncle.
- (Corcos et al)

S. S. Goonewardene et al., *Basic Urological Management*,
https://doi.org/10.1007/978-3-319-98720-0_95

History

- Frquency, urgency, nocturia, (storage symtptoms).
- Weak stream, straining, hesitancy, terminal dribbling (voiding symptoms).
- Associated haematuria, UTIS, or incontinence.
- When did the symptoms start, extent and duration.
- Past medical history and medicines.
- Bowel and gynaecological history-any episiotomies or tears.
- Neurological or medical conditions.
- Smoking.
- (Gormley et al)

Examination

- Assess the abdomen: palpable bladder?
- If female, PV examination-evidence of atrophic vaginitis, cystocoele, ureterocoele, pelvic masses, rectal prolapse.
- If male, DRE-size, consistency and regularity of prostate.

Investigations

- Urine dip and culture-rule out haematuria, and UTIS.
- Flow rate-to assess the rate of bladder emptying, voided volume and PVR.
- Bladder diary-to assess fluid intake, symptoms experienced and voided volume.
- USS KUB-stones?, any bladder masses?
- Flexible cystoscopy-any bladder tumours, CIS.

Management

- Conservative management: bladder diary, weight loss, cut out caffeine, bladder retraining, PFE, stop smoking.
- 1st line medical therapy-oxybutinin, solifancin, tolteradine. (Jayarajan et al)
- Mirabegron (B3 agonist), then conbination therapy with one of the above.
- If medical therapy fails, urodynamic analysis prior to operative intervention
- Patients may not comply with medical therapy due to the side effect profile (Tae Heon Kim).
- Then intravesical botox injections into the bladder (trigone sparing).
- If this fails, for referral to a specialist centre for neuromodulation, then clam augmentation cystoplasty if appropriate.

Suggested Reading

Corcos J, Przydacz M, Campeau L, Witten J, Hickling D, Honeine C, Radomski SB, Stothers L, Wagg A. CUA guideline on adult overactive bladder. Can Urol Assoc J. 2017;11(5):E142–73.

Gormley EA, Lightner DJ, Faraday M, Vasavada SP. Diagnosis and treatment of overactive bladder (non-neurogenic) in adults: AUA/SUFU guideline amendment. J Urol. 2015;193(5):1572–80.

Jayarajan J, Radomski SB. Pharmacotherapy of overactive bladder in adults: a review of efficacy, tolerability, and quality of life. Res Rep Urol. 2014;6:1–16.

Kim TH, Lee K-S. Persistence and compliance with medication management in the treatment of overactive bladder. Investig Clin Urol. 2016;57(2):84–93.

Diagnosis of Overactive Bladder

96

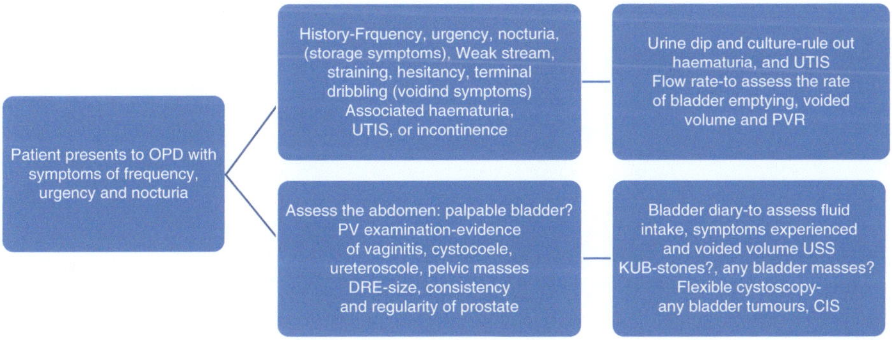

Suggested Reading

Corcos J, Przydacz M, Campeau L, Witten J, Hickling D, Honeine C, Radomski SB, Stothers L, Wagg A. CUA guideline on adult overactive bladder. Can Urol Assoc J. 2017;11(5):E142–73.

Gormley EA, Lightner DJ, Faraday M, Vasavada SP. Diagnosis and treatment of overactive bladder (non-neurogenic) in adults: AUA/SUFU guideline amendment. J Urol. 2015;193(5):1572–80.

Jayarajan J, Radomski SB. Pharmacotherapy of overactive bladder in adults: a review of efficacy, tolerability, and quality of life. Res Rep Urol. 2014;6:1–16.

Kim TH, Lee K-S. Persistence and compliance with medication management in the treatment of overactive bladder. Investig Clin Urol. 2016;57(2):84–93.

S. S. Goonewardene et al., *Basic Urological Management*,
https://doi.org/10.1007/978-3-319-98720-0_96

Management of Overactive Bladder

97

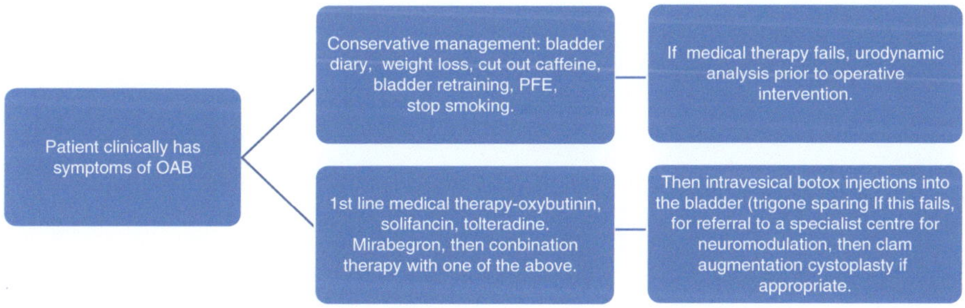

Suggested Reading

Corcos J, Przydacz M, Campeau L, Witten J, Hickling D, Honeine C, Radomski SB, Stothers L, Wagg A. CUA guideline on adult overactive bladder. Can Urol Assoc J. 2017;11(5):E142–73.

Gormley EA, Lightner DJ, Faraday M, Vasavada SP. Diagnosis and treatment of overactive bladder (non-neurogenic) in adults: AUA/SUFU guideline amendment. J Urol. 2015;193(5):1572–80.

Jayarajan J, Radomski SB. Pharmacotherapy of overactive bladder in adults: a review of efficacy, tolerability, and quality of life. Res Rep Urol. 2014;6:1–16.

Kim TH, Lee K-S. Persistence and compliance with medication management in the treatment of overactive bladder. Investig Clin Urol. 2016;57(2):84–93.

S. S. Goonewardene et al., *Basic Urological Management*,
https://doi.org/10.1007/978-3-319-98720-0_97

Urinary Incontinence

98

Definition

- Involuntary leakage of urine in a socially unacceptable place.
- Stress incontinence-leakage on coughing, sneezing, increased abdominal pressure.
- Urge incontinence-leakage with associated urgency.
- Urinary incontinence maybe stress incontinence, urge incontinence or mixed incontinence.
- There are different paths of management depending on type.

Causes

- Stress incontinence: childbirth (episiotomies), forceps delivery (damage to external sphincter).
- Urge incontinence-leakage with associated urgency.
- Mixed incontinence.

S. S. Goonewardene et al., *Basic Urological Management*,
https://doi.org/10.1007/978-3-319-98720-0_98

History

- Extent and duration of symptoms-ICIQ-SF questionnaire.
- Exacerbation and progession.
- LUTS, UTIS, haematuria.
- Leakage episodes, pad weight, changes of clothing.
- Associated bowel and gynaecological history.
- (NICE Guidelines, CG171).

Examination

- Review the abdomen:
- Palpable bladder (?retention or high post void residuals),
- Masses in flanks.
- General abdominal examination, alsod looking for abdominal pathology, constipation, obstruction.
- PV examination (chapteroned): leakage on cough test from urethra atrophic vaginitis, cystocoele, ureterocoele, rectocoele.

Investigation

- Urine dip and culture, flows.
- USS KUB and PVR-do they have other pathology (stones, obstructive uropathy) or a urethral stricture?
- Bladder diary, ICIQ and Quality of life questionnaires.
- Flexible cystoscopy-rule out a bladder tumour.
- Urodynamics-prior to surgery.
- (Burkhard et al)

Management

- Stress incontinence-conservative measures, weight loss, PFE exercises with a physiothreapist.
- TVT, TOT or bulking agents (Ellington et al).
- Urge incontinence-conservative measures, cut out caffeine.
- Medical therapy-oxybutinin, solifenacin, tolteradine
- Operative measure-botox injections, neuromodulation.
- Mixed incontinence-urodynamics to determine which symptoms are more bothersome then treat more bothersome.

Suggested Reading

Burkhard FC, Bosch JLHR, Cruz F, Lemack GE, Nambiar AK, Thiruchelvam N, Tubaro A. Guidelines Associates: Ambühl D, Bedretdinova D, Farag F, Lombardo R, Schneider MP. EAU guidelines on urinary incontinence. 2018.

Ellington DR, Erekson EA, Richter HE. Outcomes of surgery for stress urinary incontinence in the older woman. Clin Geriatr Med. 2015;31(4):487–505.

NICE Guidelines CG 171, 2013.

Diagnosis of Incontinence

99

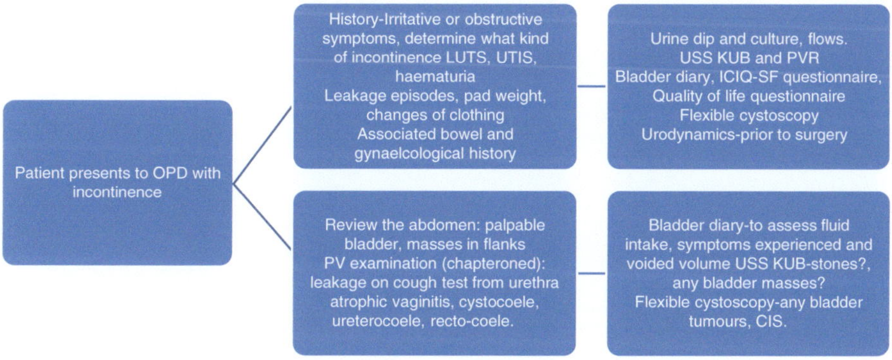

Suggested Reading

Burkhard FC, Bosch JLHR, Cruz F, Lemack GE, Nambiar AK, Thiruchelvam N, Tubaro A. Guidelines Associates: Ambühl D, Bedretdinova D, Farag F, Lombardo R, Schneider MP. EAU guidelines on urinary incontinence. 2018.

Ellington DR, Erekson EA, Richter HE. Outcomes of surgery for stress urinary incontinence in the older woman. Clin Geriatr Med. 2015;31(4):487–505.

NICE Guidelines CG 171, 2013.

S. S. Goonewardene et al., *Basic Urological Management*,
https://doi.org/10.1007/978-3-319-98720-0_99

Management of Incontinence

100

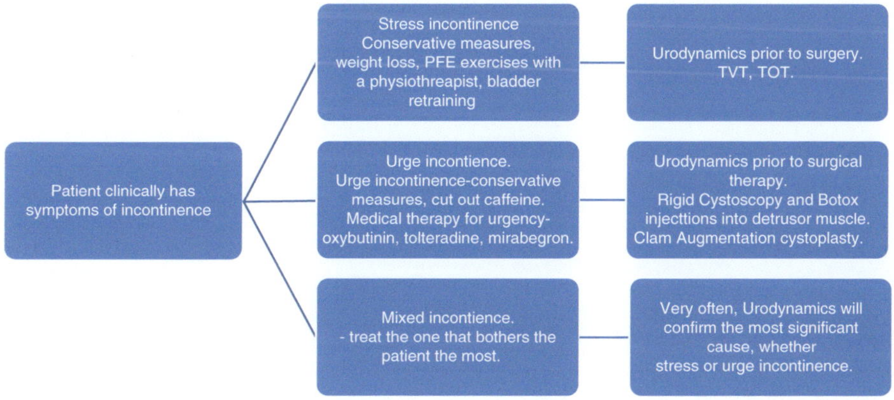

Suggested Reading

Burkhard FC, Bosch JLHR, Cruz F, Lemack GE, Nambiar AK, Thiruchelvam N, Tubaro A. Guidelines Associates: Ambühl D, Bedretdinova D, Farag F, Lombardo R, Schneider MP. EAU guidelines on urinary incontinence. 2018.

Ellington DR, Erekson EA, Richter HE. Outcomes of surgery for stress urinary incontinence in the older woman. Clin Geriatr Med. 2015;31(4):487–505.

NICE Guidelines CG 171, 2013.

S. S. Goonewardene et al., *Basic Urological Management*,
https://doi.org/10.1007/978-3-319-98720-0_100

Priapism

101

Definition

- Persistence of an erection after cessation or removal of the stimulus that caused it.
- It can be painful, pulseless, and purple in colour.
- There are two types ischaemic or none ischaemic.
- It must be reversed within 6 hrs.
- Penile gangrene can be a complication (Ajape et al)
- (Babcock et al)

Causes

- Sickle cell anaemia.
- Leukaemia, lymphoma, thalassaemia.
- Glucose 6 phosphate deficiency.
- Intracaversal injections- alprostadil, caverject.
- Drugs- cocaine, chlorpromazine, clozapine.
- Spinal cord injury.
- Prostate cancer.

S. S. Goonewardene et al., *Basic Urological Management*,
https://doi.org/10.1007/978-3-319-98720-0_101

History

- Extent and duration of symptoms.
- Exacerbating factotrs. prior history or shunts.
- LUTS, UTIS, haematuria.
- Any drugs taken, anything applied to penis, foreign bodies eg penile rings etc.

Examination

- Examination of the abdomen, general medical exam
- Examination and grading of erection.
- Assess general fitness for anaesthetic.

Investigations

- Bloods inc WCC, crp, Renal functions, sickle cell screen, clotting.
- Blood gas from penis- is it ischaemic or none ischaemic.

Management

- Conservative measures- running up and down stairs, ice packs.
- Medical interventions
- Venflow- orange into each corpora bilaterally- blood aspirated (400 ml) and flush through with saline
- Take ABG of blood sample to determine if ischaemic or none ischaemic.
- If none ischaemic, use 0.1 ml of phenylephrine in 10 ml saline under cardiac monitoring into the corpora, instil in 50 microgram aliquots. Have an anaesthetist present.
- If fails- Winters or T shunt- using trus biopsy needle, punture each corpora.
- If ischaemic, arterial embolisation.
- (Montague et al)

Suggested Reading

Ajape AA, Bello A. Penile gangrene: an unusual complication of priapism in a patient with bladder carcinoma. J Surg Tech Case Rep. 2010;3:37–9.

Babcock C. Emergency department management of priapism. Emerg Med Pract. 2017;19(1):1–16.

Montague DK, Jarow J, Broderick GA, Dmochowski RR, Heaton JP, Lue TF, Nehra A, Sharlip ID. American Urological Association guideline on the management of priapism. J Urol. 2003;170(4 Pt 1):1318–24.

Diagnosis of Priapism

102

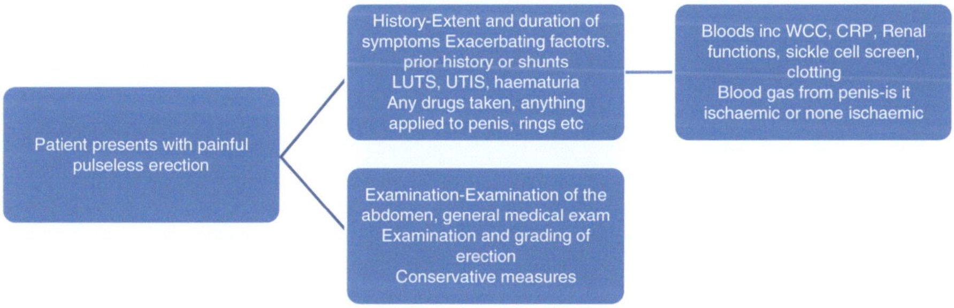

Suggested Reading

Ajape AA, Bello A. Penile gangrene: an unusual complication of priapism in a patient with bladder carcinoma. J Surg Tech Case Rep. 2010;3:37–9.

Babcock C. Emergency department management of priapism. Emerg Med Pract. 2017;19(1):1–16.

Montague DK, Jarow J, Broderick GA, Dmochowski RR, Heaton JP, Lue TF, Nehra A, Sharlip ID. American Urological Association guideline on the management of priapism. J Urol. 2003;170(4 Pt 1):1318–24.

S. S. Goonewardene et al., *Basic Urological Management*,
https://doi.org/10.1007/978-3-319-98720-0_102

Management of Priapism

103

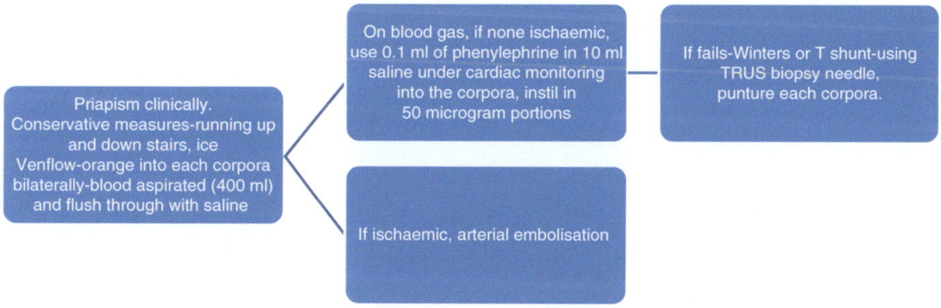

Suggested Reading

Ajape AA, Bello A. Penile gangrene: an unusual complication of priapism in a patient with bladder carcinoma. J Surg Tech Case Rep. 2010;3:37–9.

Babcock C. Emergency department management of priapism. Emerg Med Pract. 2017;19(1):1–16.

Montague DK, Jarow J, Broderick GA, Dmochowski RR, Heaton JP, Lue TF, Nehra A, Sharlip ID. American Urological Association guideline on the management of priapism. J Urol. 2003;170(4 Pt 1):1318–24.

S. S. Goonewardene et al., *Basic Urological Management*,
https://doi.org/10.1007/978-3-319-98720-0_103

Penile Fracture

104

Definition

- Rupture of Bucks fascia that envelopes the corpora cavernosa with or without associated urethral injury.
- If there is haemturia there is associated urethral injury.
- Urethral injury may be complete or partial.
- Requires operative intervention to fix rupture.
- (Haas et al)

Causes

- Intercourse where pressure is put on penis.
- Aggressive masturbation.
- Results in rupture of bucks fascia with involvement of the tunica.

S. S. Goonewardene et al., *Basic Urological Management*,
https://doi.org/10.1007/978-3-319-98720-0_104

History

- Extent and duration of symptoms
- Time of injury, time since injury
- Haematuria
- Any popping sound
- Pain
- Immediate detumesence
- Blood at the urethral meatus, retention
- (Mirzazadeh et al)

Examination

- Review the abdomen: palpable bladder? retention.
- Blood at external urethral meatus? (urethral injury)
- Is there a palpable defect-break in Bucks fascia
- Egg plant sign-swollen bruised penis, painful.

Invstigation

- Urine dip and culture.
- Bloods-FBC, U+Es, Clotting, G+S.
- USS penis or MRI penis (to look for break in tunica). Saglan et al, Merjadi et al.

Management

- Surgical exploration and repair.
- Consent to include circumcision, degloving of penile skin to base, identification and evacuation of haematoma and repair of defect in bucks fascia-consent should also include on table urethogram and repair of urethral injury.
- Catheterise patient as part of procedure.

Suggested Reading

Haas CA, Brown SL, Spirnak JP. Penile fracture and testicular rupture. World J Urol. 1999;17(2):101–6.

Mirzazadeh M, Fallahkarkan M, Hosseini J. Penile fracture epidemiology, diagnosis and management in Iran: a narrative review. Transl Androl Urol. 2017;6(2):158–66.

Saglam E, Tarhan F, Hamarat MB, Can U, Coskun A, Camur E, Sarica K. Efficacy of magnetic resonance imaging for diagnosis of penile fracture: a controlled study. Investig Clin Urol. 2017;58(4):255–60.

Zare MM, Darabi M, Bagheri SM, Kamali K, Bijan B. The role of ultrasound (US) and magnetic resonance imaging (MRI) in penile fracture mapping for modified surgical repair. Int Urol Nephrol. 2017;49(6):937–45.

105 Diagnosis of Penile Fracture

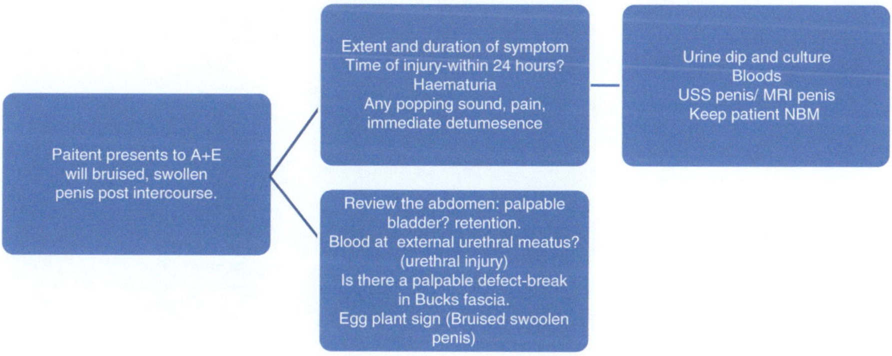

S. S. Goonewardene et al., *Basic Urological Management*,
https://doi.org/10.1007/978-3-319-98720-0_105

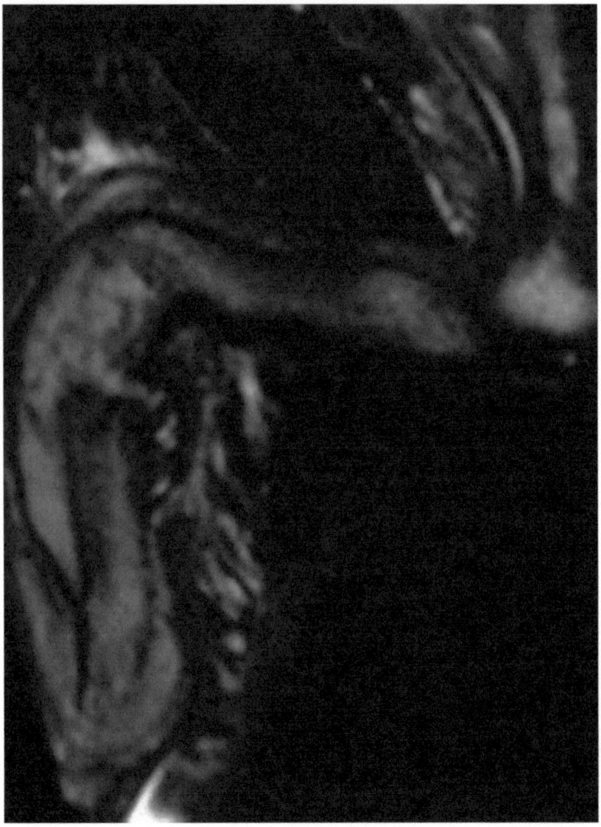

Fig. 105.1 MRI demonstrating penile fracture

Suggested Reading

Haas CA, Brown SL, Spirnak JP. Penile fracture and testicular rupture. World J Urol. 1999;17(2):101–6.

Mirzazadeh M, Fallahkarkan M, Hosseini J. Penile fracture epidemiology, diagnosis and management in Iran: a narrative review. Transl Androl Urol. 2017;6(2):158–66.

Saglam E, Tarhan F, Hamarat MB, Can U, Coskun A, Camur E, Sarica K. Efficacy of magnetic resonance imaging for diagnosis of penile fracture: a controlled study. Investig Clin Urol. 2017;58(4):255–60.

Zare MM, Darabi M, Bagheri SM, Kamali K, Bijan B. The role of ultrasound (US) and magnetic resonance imaging (MRI) in penile fracture mapping for modified surgical repair. Int Urol Nephrol. 2017;49(6):937–45.

Management of Penile Fracture

106

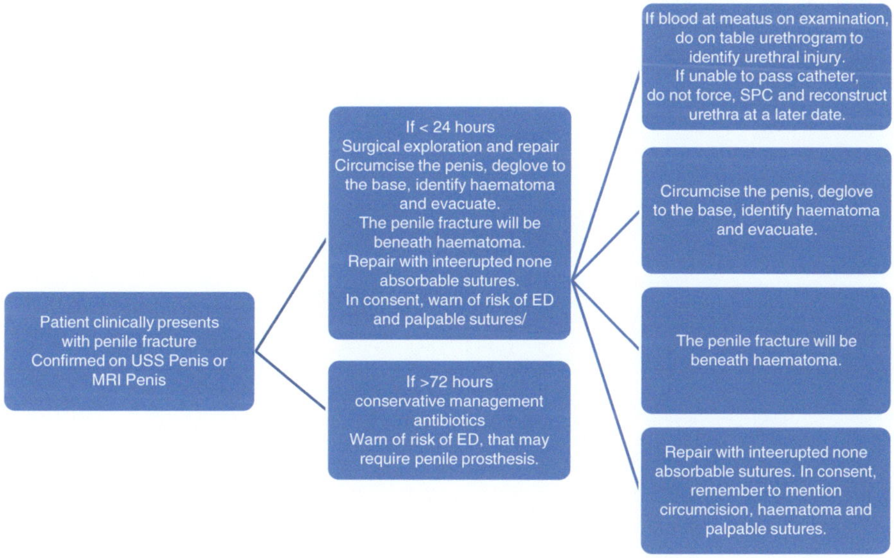

S. S. Goonewardene et al., *Basic Urological Management*,
https://doi.org/10.1007/978-3-319-98720-0_106

Suggested Reading

Haas CA, Brown SL, Spirnak JP. Penile fracture and testicular rupture. World J Urol. 1999;17(2):101–6.

Mirzazadeh M, Fallahkarkan M, Hosseini J. Penile fracture epidemiology, diagnosis and management in Iran: a narrative review. Transl Androl Urol. 2017;6(2):158–66.

Saglam E, Tarhan F, Hamarat MB, Can U, Coskun A, Camur E, Sarica K. Efficacy of magnetic resonance imaging for diagnosis of penile fracture: a controlled study. Investig Clin Urol. 2017;58(4):255–60.

Zare MM, Darabi M, Bagheri SM, Kamali K, Bijan B. The role of ultrasound (US) and magnetic resonance imaging (MRI) in penile fracture mapping for modified surgical repair. Int Urol Nephrol. 2017;49(6):937–45.

107 Phimosis

Definition

- Inability to retract foreskin.
- Tightening of foreskin on retraction around glans.
- Usually caused by BXO.
- Can often result in poor penile hygiene.

Causes

- Diabetes mellitus.
- BXO, thickened tight foreskin.
- Paediatric phimosis can occur, but do not confuse with physiological phimosis, where the foreskin has not fully developed yet (this should have occured by the age of 5).

S. S. Goonewardene et al., *Basic Urological Management*,
https://doi.org/10.1007/978-3-319-98720-0_107

History

- Extent and duration of symptoms.
- Exacerbation-ripping, tearing and healing multiple times.
- Bleedng from torn foreskins.
- No LUTS, UTIS-check for retention.
- Past medical history DM, BXO treatment, steroids.

Examination

- Review the abdomen: palpable bladder, masses in flanks.
- Examine external genitalia for any masses (penile tumour).
- Get the patient to retract the foreskin back as far as they can-it is important to let them do this as it is painful on retraction.
- Some may not be able to retract at all, as the foreskin will be plastered to the glans.

Invstigation

- Urine dip and culture
- Uroflowetry
- Bloods

Management

- If phimosis is present, and the patient is voiding, list for a circumcision under GA-especially in cases where the foreskin is none retractile, it can be a difficult dissection.
- Counsel the patient for complications of cirumcision including poor cosmesis, penile curvature, glans sensivitity. wound complications, decreased sensation, decreased orgasmic sensation.
- In most cases like this a frenuoplasty will not work-the foreskin is tight and will not be relieved by a frenuloplasty.
- THere is no such thing as a partial circumcision.

Suggested Reading

Lee CH, Lee SD. Effect of topical steroid (0.05% clobetasol propionate) treatment in children with severe phimosis. Korean J Urol. 2013;54(9):624–30.

McGregor TB, Pike JG, Leonard MP. Pathologic and physiologic phimosis: approach to the phimotic foreskin. Can Fam Physician. 2007;53(3):445–8.

Wilson WR. Phimosis. Br Med J. 1956;1(4978):1279.

Diagnosis and Management of Phimosis

108

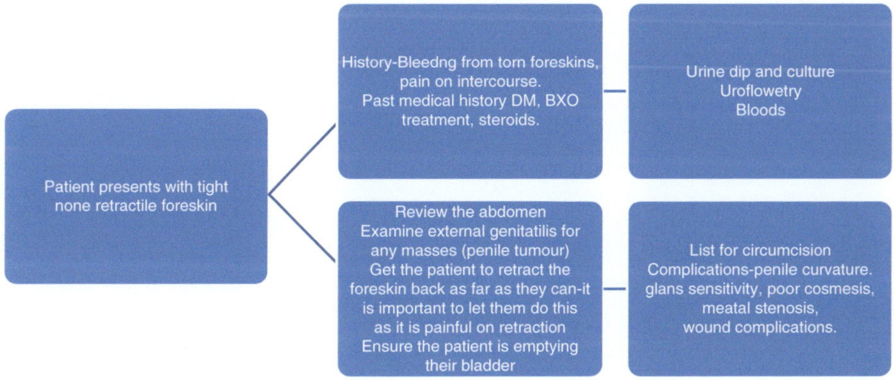

Suggested Reading

Lee CH, Lee SD. Effect of topical steroid (0.05% clobetasol propionate) treatment in children with severe phimosis. Korean J Urol. 2013;54(9):624–30.

McGregor TB, Pike JG, Leonard MP. Pathologic and physiologic phimosis: approach to the phimotic foreskin. Can Fam Physician. 2007;53(3):445–8.

Wilson WR. Phimosis. Br Med J. 1956;1(4978):1279.

S. S. Goonewardene et al., *Basic Urological Management*,
https://doi.org/10.1007/978-3-319-98720-0_108

109 Paraphimosis

Definition

- Inablity to retract foreskin due to swelling and oedema of the distal penile skin due to constriction.
- Often caused by the foreskin being retracted and not being replaced.
- It is a time critical event-the longer it remained unreduced, the more diffcult it will be to reduce. (Olsen et al)

Causes

- None replacement of foreskin into normal anatomical position.
- E.g. post catheterisation, post intercourse.
- If prolonged, it can lead to gangrene, penile necrosis and amputation.

S. S. Goonewardene et al., *Basic Urological Management*,
https://doi.org/10.1007/978-3-319-98720-0_109

History

- Extent and duration of symptoms.
- Pain, LUTS, UTIS.
- Prior paraphimosis and reduction.
- Any attempt at reduction.

Examination

- Review the abdomen: palpable bladder?
- Examine the penis for masses.
- If the foreskin is retracted, assess extent and degree.

Invstigation

- Urine dip and culture
- Uroflowmetry
- Bloods

Management

- Penile block-2% lidocaine without adrenaline in a circumferential block around penile base and to penile nerves (inject behind symphisis pubis).
- Atttempt manual reduction-firm compression for reduction over 30 mins using palms of both hands-also try to pull the foreskin upwards.
- If fails try 20% dextrose solution and needle punctures to swollen area to reduce.
- If that fails, list for dorsal slit +/–circumcision under GA
- (Mackway-Jones et al, Yutaro et al).

Suggested Reading

Hayashi Y, Kojima Y, Mizuno K, Kohri K. Prepuce: phimosis, paraphimosis, and circumcision. Sci World J. 2011;11:289–301.

Mackway-Jones K, Teece S. Ice, pins, or sugar to reduce paraphimosis. Emerg Med J. 2004;21(1):77–8.

Olson C. Emergency treatment of paraphimosis. Can Fam Physician. 1998;44:1253–4, 1257.

Management of Paraphimosis

110

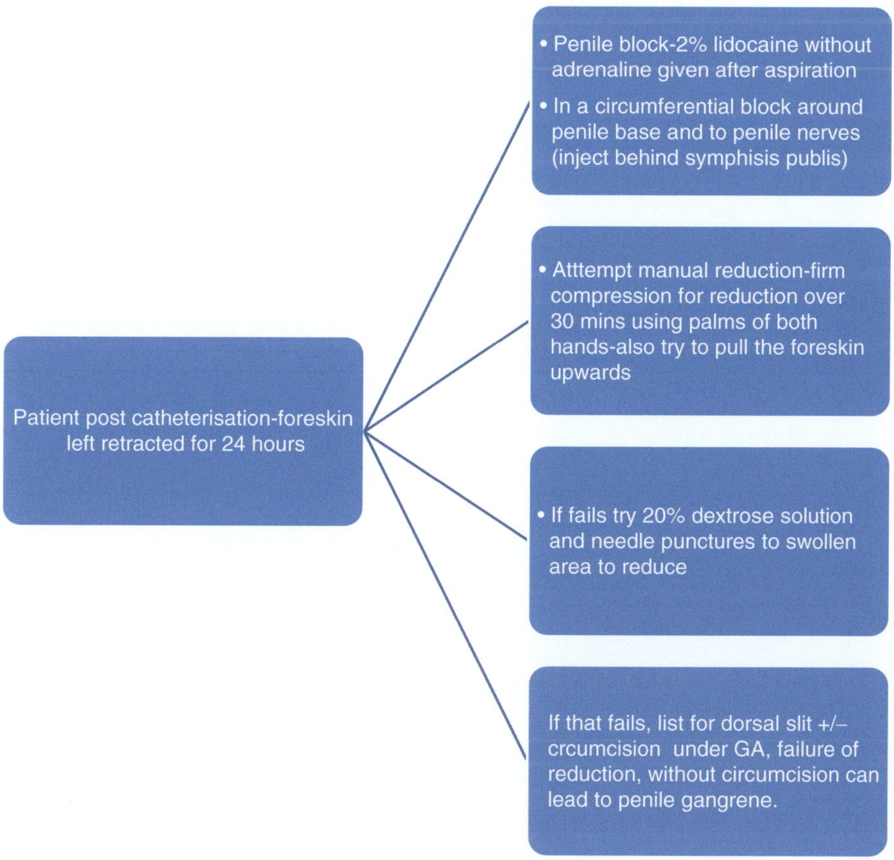

S. S. Goonewardene et al., *Basic Urological Management*,
https://doi.org/10.1007/978-3-319-98720-0_110

Suggested Reading

Hayashi Y, Kojima Y, Mizuno K, Kohri K. Prepuce: phimosis, paraphimosis, and circumcision. Sci World J. 2011;11:289–301.

Mackway-Jones K, Teece S. Ice, pins, or sugar to reduce paraphimosis. Emerg Med J. 2004;21(1):77–8.

Olson C. Emergency treatment of paraphimosis. Can Fam Physician. 1998;44:1253–4, 1257.

Erectile Dysfunction

111

Definition

- Inablity to get an erection.
- Erection not sufficient for intercourse.
- Unable to complete intercourse satisfactorily.

Causes

- Diabetes.
- Cardiac disease-angiopaths, renal and liver disease.
- Obesity, high cholesterol, high BP.
- Neuropathic disease, neurogenic disorders.
- Medication: tamsulosin.
- Psychological disorders.
- Post operatve, post radical prostatectomy, post turp
- (Faysal et al), (Banks et al)

S. S. Goonewardene et al., *Basic Urological Management*,
https://doi.org/10.1007/978-3-319-98720-0_111

History

- Grade erection-IIEF/SHIM Score.
- Extent and duration of symptoms.
- Nocturnal erections, general fitness (DM, cardiac, respiratory, liver or renal disease), other co-morbidities.
- Prior therapy and assessment.
- If post op-what procedure.
- History of neuropathy?

Examination

- Obs-blood pressure, heart reate, respiratory rate.
- Assessment of vascular disease.
- Examination of abdomen.
- Assessment of scrotum and testicular size (good sized testicles?) and presence of varicoeles.
- Penile assessment-penile plaques.
- ? General fitness and elevated BMI?
- Any neurological defect.
- DRE-prostate cancer present?

Invstigation

- Bloods: TFTs, Testosterone, LH, FSH, SHBG, U+Es, glucose, PSA.
- USS Testes-to assess for underlying pathology.
- Urine dip and culture.

Management

- PDE 5 inhibitors, viagra, levitra, tadafil.
- Vacuum pump device.
- Follow-up in an andrology clinic.
- 2nd line-caverject-alprostadil injection into corpora of penis or MUSE (intraurethral capsule).
- If these measures fail, consider penile prosthesis.
- (Pastuszak et al)

Suggested Reading

Banks E, Joshy G, Abhayaratna WP, Kritharides L, Macdonald PS, Korda RJ, Chalmers JP. Erectile dysfunction severity as a risk marker for cardiovascular disease hospitalisation and all-cause mortality: a prospective cohort study. PLoS Med. 2013;10(1):e1001372.

Pastuszak AW. Current diagnosis and management of erectile dysfunction. Curr Sex Health Rep. 2014;6(3):164–76.

Yafi FA, Jenkins L, Albersen M, Corona G, Isidori AM, Goldfarb S, Maggi M, Nelson CJ, Parish S, Salonia A, Tan R, Mulhall JP, Hellstrom WJG. Erectile dysfunction. Nat Rev Dis Primers. 2016;2:16003.

Diagnosis and Management of ED

112

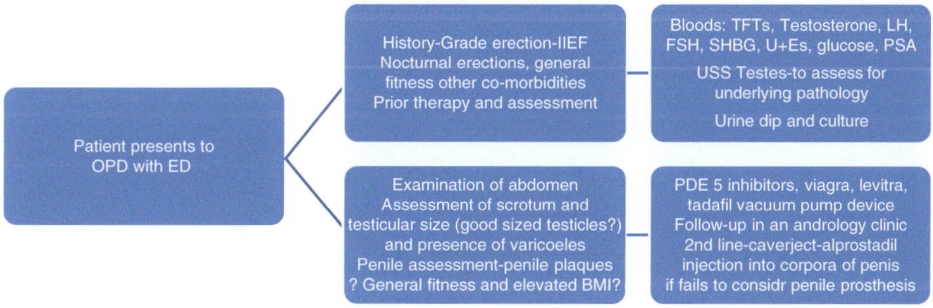

Suggested Reading

Banks E, Joshy G, Abhayaratna WP, Kritharides L, Macdonald PS, Korda RJ, Chalmers JP. Erectile dysfunction severity as a risk marker for cardiovascular disease hospitalisation and all-cause mortality: a prospective cohort study. PLoS Med. 2013;10(1):e1001372.

Pastuszak AW. Current diagnosis and management of erectile dysfunction. Curr Sex Health Rep. 2014;6(3):164–76.

Yafi FA, Jenkins L, Albersen M, Corona G, Isidori AM, Goldfarb S, Maggi M, Nelson CJ, Parish S, Salonia A, Tan R, Mulhall JP, Hellstrom WJG. Erectile dysfunction. Nat Rev Dis Primers. 2016;2:16003.

S. S. Goonewardene et al., *Basic Urological Management*,
https://doi.org/10.1007/978-3-319-98720-0_112

113 Penile Cancer

Definition

- Presence of SCC in the penis.
- Due to a number of factors including presence of a foreskin.
- Organ sparing surgery is best, if the cancer stage allows.

Causes

- Presence of foreskin.
- Poor penile hygeiene.
- Smegma.
- UV radiation.
- HPV types 16 and 18.
- (Hakenberg et al)

S. S. Goonewardene et al., *Basic Urological Management*,
https://doi.org/10.1007/978-3-319-98720-0_113

History

- Lesion.
- Extent duration.
- Ulceration, skin abnormality.
- Lumps in groin.
- Past circumsions.
- Exposure to causative factors.

Examination

- Obs
- Chest, Abdominal examination.
- Presence of lesion on penis-depth of invasion and location-glans only, corpora, urethra, groin.
- Examination of groin for invasion and lymph nodes.

Invstigation

- MRI pelvis including groin and abdomen.
- Urine dipstick.

Management

- If superficial disease, glansectomy and glansoplasty or CO_2 laser and biopsy-Ta, TIS.
- If invading glans only, for partial penectomy
- If in the body of the penis invading the urethra, for penectomy and perineal urethrostomy.
- Hakkanson et al, Shabbir et al.

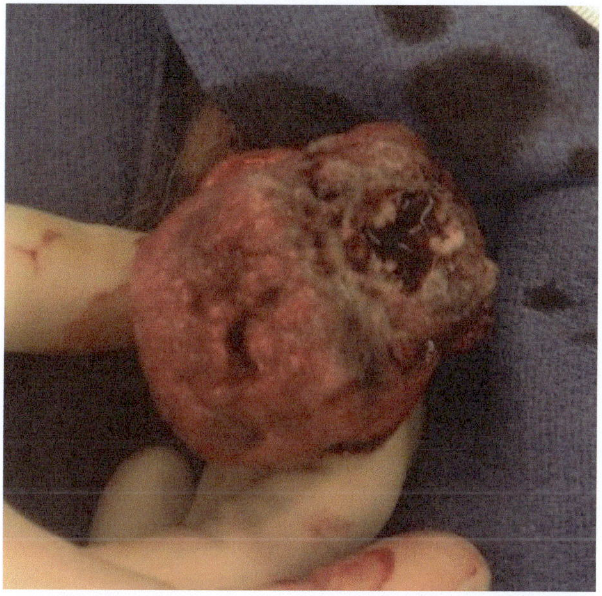

Fig. 113.1 Demonstrating penile cancer on glans

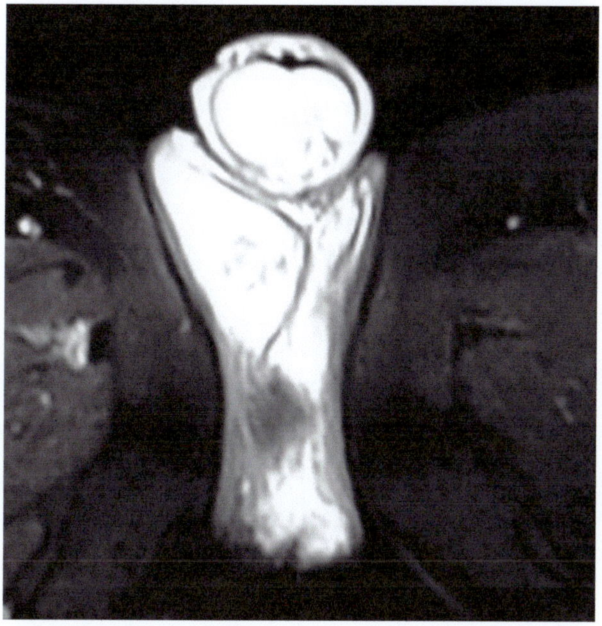

Fig. 113.2 MRI demonstrating penile cancer

Suggested Reading

Håkansson U, Kirrander P, Uvelius B, Baseckas G, Torbrand C. Organ-sparing reconstructive surgery in penile cancer: initial experiences at two Swedish referral centres. Scand J Urol. 2015;49(2):149–54.

Hakenberg OW, Compérat E, Minhas S, Necchi A, Protzel C, Watkin N, Guidelines Associate: Robinson R. EAU guidelines on penile cancer: 2014 update. Eur Urol. 2015;67(1):142–50.

Shabbir M, Kayes O, Minhas S. Challenges and controversies in the management of penile cancer. Nat Rev Urol. 2014;11(12):702–11.

Diagnosis of Penile Cancer

114

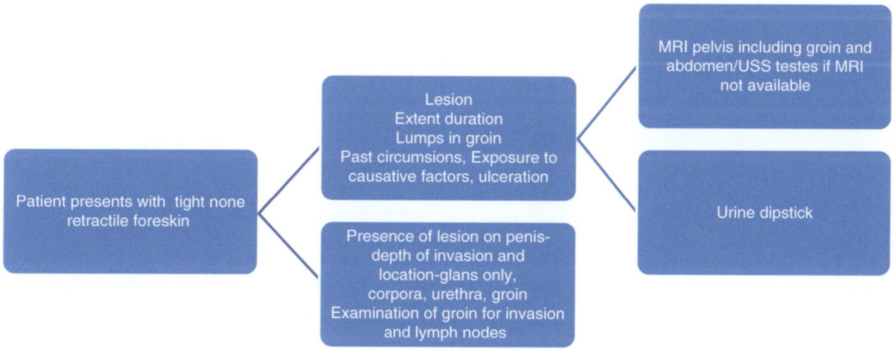

Suggested Reading

Håkansson U, Kirrander P, Uvelius B, Baseckas G, Torbrand C. Organ-sparing reconstructive surgery in penile cancer: initial experiences at two Swedish referral centres. Scand J Urol. 2015;49(2):149–54.

Hakenberg OW, Compérat E, Minhas S, Necchi A, Protzel C, Watkin N, Guidelines Associate: Robinson R. EAU guidelines on penile cancer: 2014 update. Eur Urol. 2015;67(1):142–50.

Shabbir M, Kayes O, Minhas S. Challenges and controversies in the management of penile cancer. Nat Rev Urol. 2014;11(12):702–11.

S. S. Goonewardene et al., *Basic Urological Management*,
https://doi.org/10.1007/978-3-319-98720-0_114

115 Management of Penile Cancer

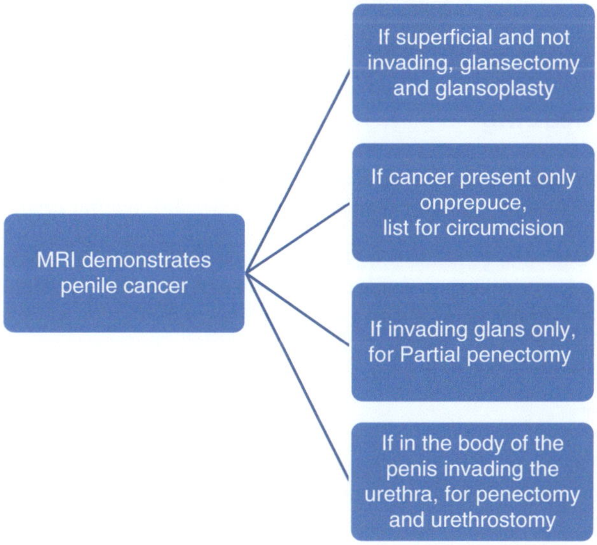

S. S. Goonewardene et al., *Basic Urological Management*,
https://doi.org/10.1007/978-3-319-98720-0_115

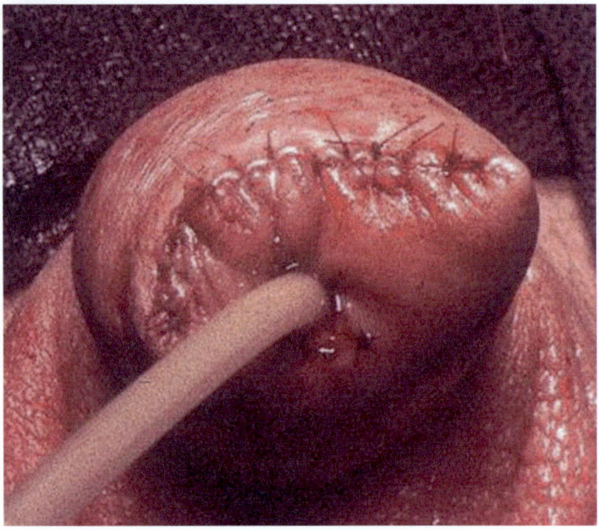

Fig. 115.1 Surgical appearance after partial penectomy

Suggested Reading

Håkansson U, Kirrander P, Uvelius B, Baseckas G, Torbrand C. Organ-sparing reconstructive surgery in penile cancer: initial experiences at two Swedish referral centres. Scand J Urol. 2015;49(2):149–54.

Hakenberg OW, Compérat E, Minhas S, Necchi A, Protzel C, Watkin N, Guidelines Associate: Robinson R. EAU guidelines on penile cancer: 2014 update. Eur Urol. 2015;67(1):142–50.

Shabbir M, Kayes O, Minhas S. Challenges and controversies in the management of penile cancer. Nat Rev Urol. 2014;11(12):702–11.

116 A Renal Mass

Definition

- A mass withith the kidney that may be benign or malign
- Renal tumours are very often picked up as incidentalomas
- Patients may present with clot colic
- Renal masses can be biopsied to determine benign or malign nature. (EAU Guidelines)

Causes

- Oncocytoma
- Renal cell Carcinoma,
- TCC of the renal pelvis
- Renal cysts
- Renal Abcess
- Staghorn calculi
- None functioning kidney

S. S. Goonewardene et al., *Basic Urological Management*,
https://doi.org/10.1007/978-3-319-98720-0_116

History

- Extent and duration of symptoms
- Pain
- A renal mass
- Flank pain (clot colic)
- Weight loss
- Bony aches (hypocalcaemia), respiratory symptoms (chest mets)
- Red appearance (malar flush)
- Left sided varicocoele (If tumour invades the renal vein on the left)
- (Pallwein-Prettner et al, Corcoran et al).

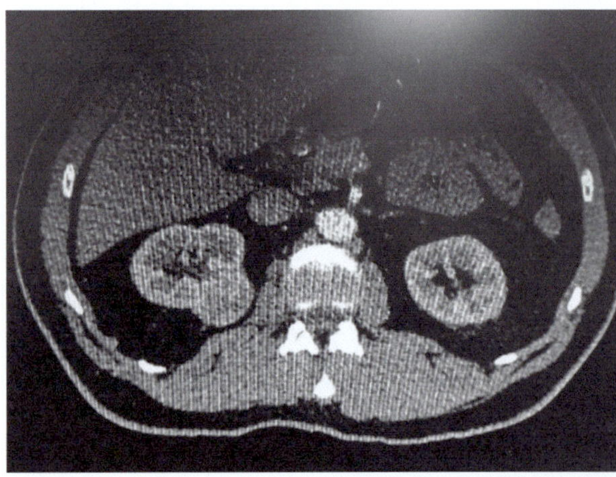

Fig. 116.1 CT demonstrating a right sided renal mass

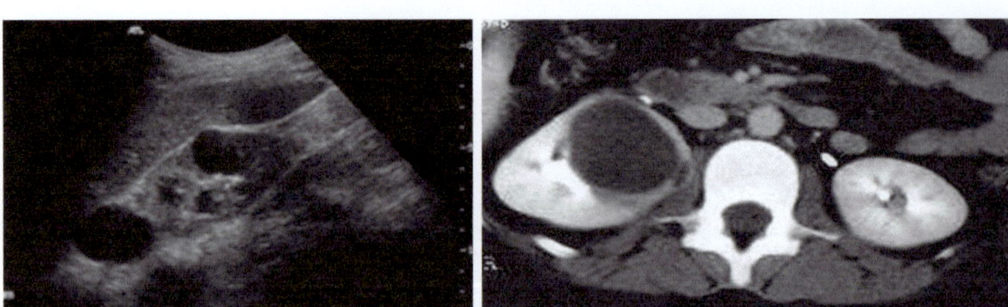

Fig. 116.2 A cystic renal mess on USS and CT

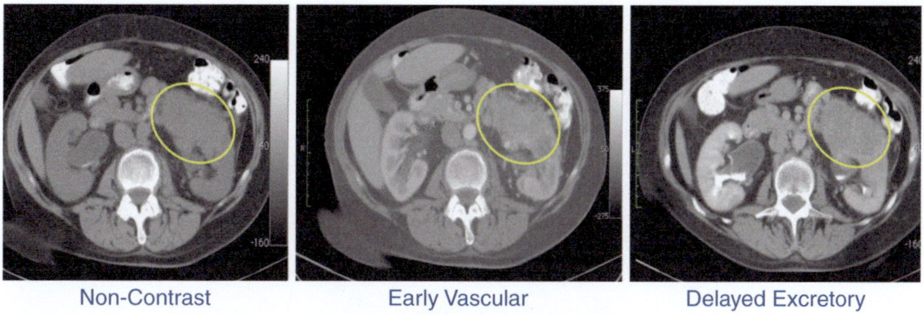

Fig. 116.3 A CT demonstrating different phases with a renal mass

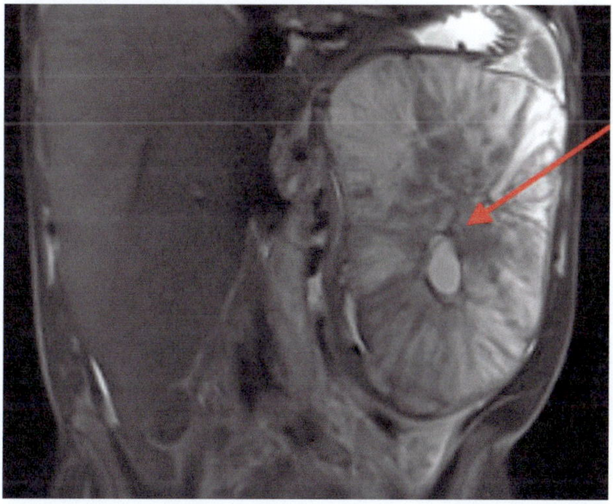

Fig. 116.4 An oncocytoma (benign renal mass) on CT

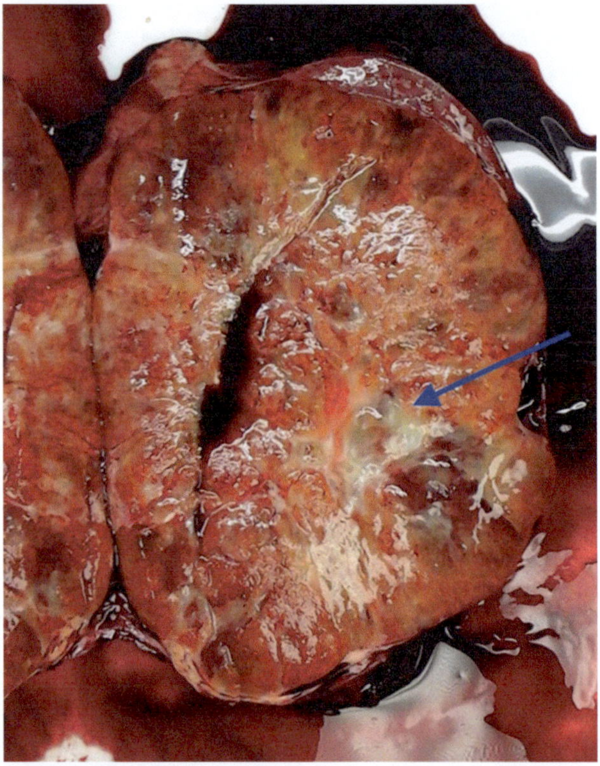

Fig. 116.5 A pathological specimen of oncocytoma

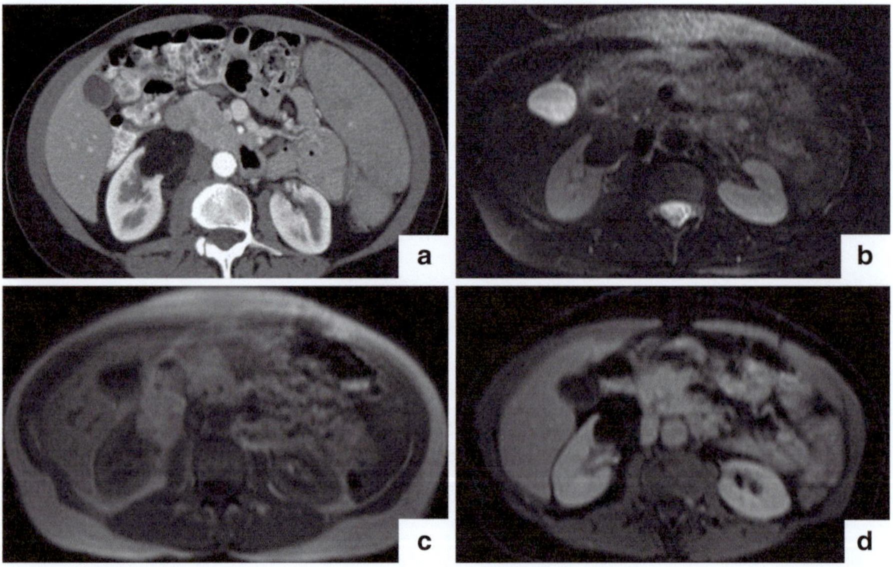

Fig. 116.6 An angiomyolipoma on CT with contrast (**a** and **b**) and none contrast (**c**–**d**) windows

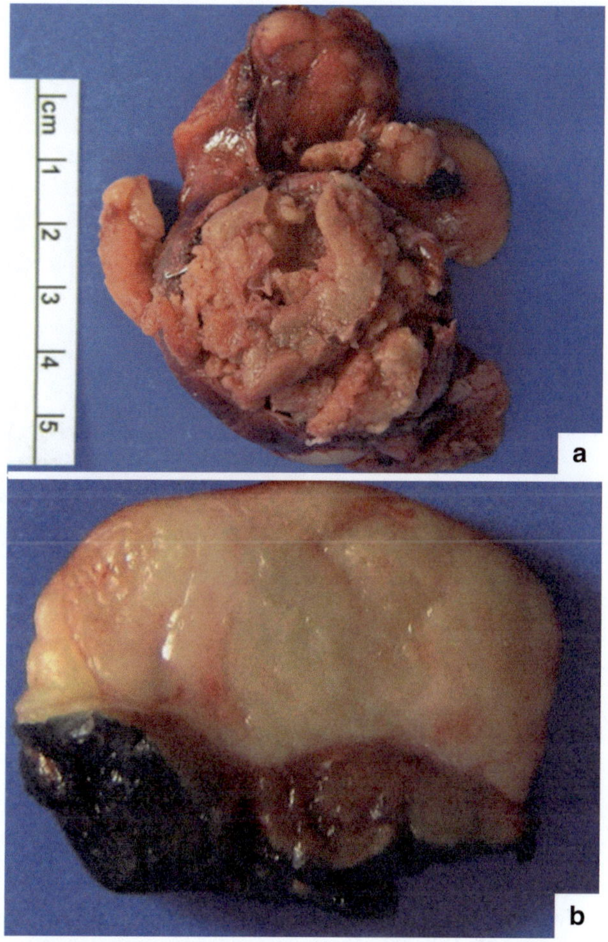

Fig. 116.7 An angiomyolipoma on pathology axial view (section **a**) and external view (section **b**)

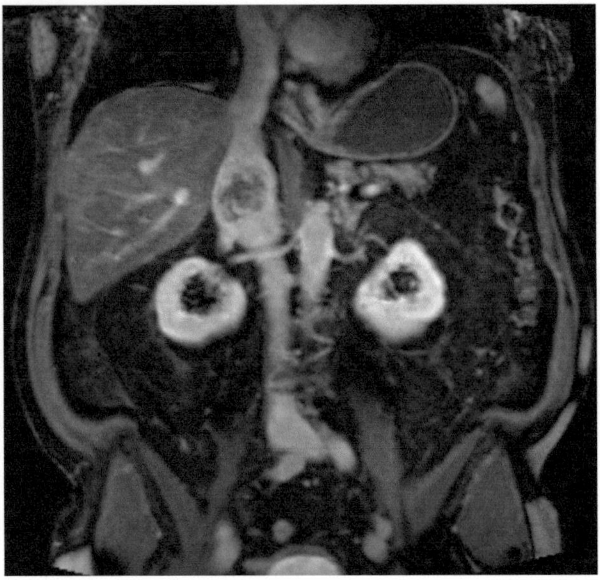

Fig. 116.8 A CT with IVC tumour thrombus with a renal RCC

Suggested Reading

Corcoran AT, Russo P, Lowrance WT, Asnis-Alibozek A, Libertino JA, Pryma DA, Divgi CR, Uzzo RG. A review of contemporary data on surgically resected renal masses—benign or malignant? Urology. 2013;81(4):707–13.

Ljungberg B, Albiges L, Bensalah K, Bex A, Giles RH, Hora M, Kuczyk MA, Lam T, Marconi L, Merseburger AS, Powles T, Staehler M, Volpe A. Guidelines Associates: Abu-Ghanem Y, Dabestani S, Fernández-Pello S, Montes, Hofmann F, Tahbaz R. EAU guidelines. Renal cell carcinoma. 2018.

Pallwein-Prettner L, Flöry D, Rotter CR, Pogner K, Syré G, Fellner C, Frauscher F, Aigner F, Krause FS, Fellner F. Assessment and characterisation of common renal masses with CT and MRI. Insights Imaging. 2011;2(5):543–56.

117 Management Pathway for Renal Mass

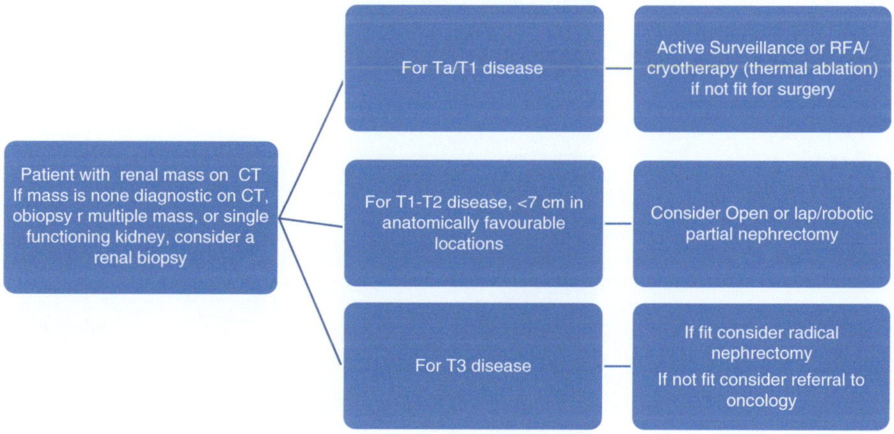

S. S. Goonewardene et al., *Basic Urological Management*,
https://doi.org/10.1007/978-3-319-98720-0_117

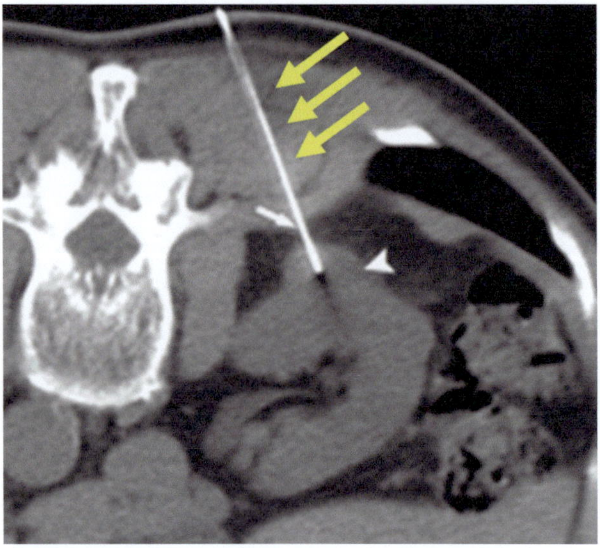

Fig. 117.1 Demonstrating percutaneous thermal ablation—CT guided

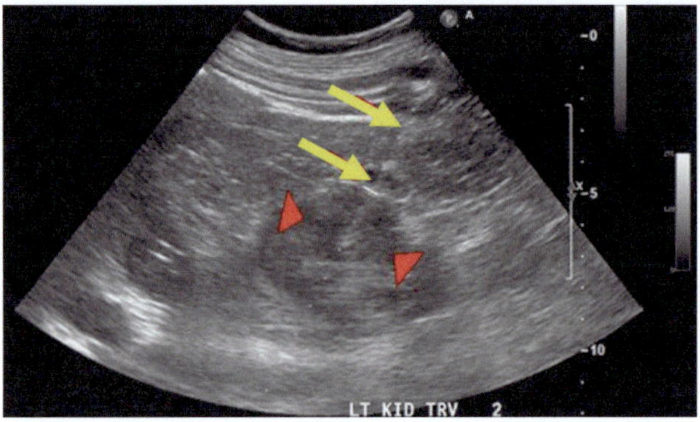

Fig. 117.2 Demonstrating renal biopsy via US guidance

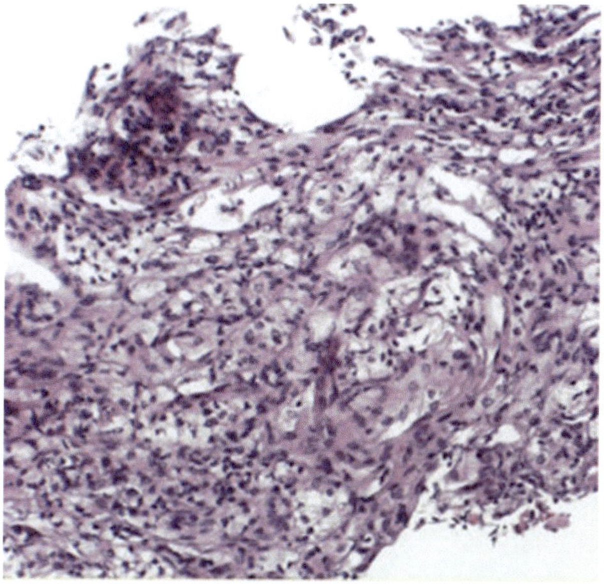

Fig. 117.3 Histology of a core biopsy from a renal mass

Suggested Reading

Corcoran AT, Russo P, Lowrance WT, Asnis-Alibozek A, Libertino JA, Pryma DA, Divgi CR, Uzzo RG. A review of contemporary data on surgically resected renal masses—benign or malignant? Urology. 2013;81(4):707–13.

Ljungberg B, Albiges L, Bensalah K, Bex A, Giles RH, Hora M, Kuczyk MA, Lam T, Marconi L, Merseburger AS, Powles T, Staehler M, Volpe A. Guidelines Associates: Abu-Ghanem Y, Dabestani S, Fernández-Pello Montes S, Hofmann F, Tahbaz R. EAU guidelines. Renal cell carcinoma. 2018.

Pallwein-Prettner L, Flöry D, Rotter CR, Pogner K, Syré G, Fellner C, Frauscher F, Aigner F, Krause FS, Fellner F. Assessment and characterisation of common renal masses with CT and MRI. Insights Imaging. 2011;2(5):543–56.

A Painful Scrotum

118

Definition

- Pain within the contents of the scrotum.
- The scrotum contains the testes, the spididymis, the spermatic cord contents including the vas, the paminiform plexus of veins, the testicular artery and artery to the vas, lymph nodes.
- Try to locailise the pain to an anatomical location.
- Be wary of torsion in the neonatal and 10-20 year old age group.
- When in doubt, explore.
- (Pogorelic et al).

Causes

- Testicular torsion
- Epididymoorchitis
- Epididymal cysts
- Hydrocoele
- Varicoele
- Necrotising fasciits
- Chronic scrotal pain
- Referred pain from the perineum

S. S. Goonewardene et al., *Basic Urological Management*,
https://doi.org/10.1007/978-3-319-98720-0_118

History

- Extent and duration of symptoms.
- Pain-when did it start? Does it radiate?
- Is it intermittent? lying higher?
- Is the testicle tender (Torsion).
- Change in appearance of the scrotum-swelling, erthyema, redness, skin changes (black or necrotic).
- Associated urinary symptoms, LUTS, dysuria, retention.
- Trauma history.
- Prior scrotal fixation .

Examination

- Obs-blood pressure, heart rate, respiratory rate.
- Assessment of abdomen-ureteric colic, appendicitis, can present as scrotal pain.
- Palpable bladder-retention.
- Examine testicles lying and standing.
- Look for normal lye, pain (localised to anatomical location), cremasteric reflex, Prehns sign (if infective cause, pain will reduce with support to testicle), cord tenderness and high lying testicle (torsion), enlarged swollen testicle (epididymo-orchitis). Transilluminate testicle (illumination-hydrocoele).

Investigation

- Bloods: FBC, renal function, crp and clotting.
- Urine dip and culture.
- USS testes if epidiymo-orchitis, hydrocoele or trauma.
- If torsion is suspected and has been present for greater than 24 hours-USS testes to see if the testicle is viable.
- (D'Andrea et al)

Management

- Testicular torsion <24 hours-surgical exploration.
- Epidiymo-orchitis-medical management-antbiotics, send off culture and scortal support-can take up to 6 weeks to resolve
- Hydrocoele-Jaboulay or Lords Plication.
- Testicular trauma-if tunica is breached on USS testes, for scrotal exploration and closure.
- Necrotising fasciits-immediate surgical debridement with General Surgical team (in case of stoma formation).
- Chronic scrotal pain-look and ensure patient is emptying badder, then refer to pain clinic.
- (Ta et al)

Suggested Reading

D'Andrea A, Coppolino F, Cesarano E, Russo A, Cappabianca S, Genovese EA, Fonio P, Macarini L. US in the assessment of acute scrotum. Crit Ultrasound J. 2013;5(Suppl 1):S8.

Pogorelić Z, Mustapić K, Jukić M, Todorić J, Mrklić I, Meštrović J, Jurić I, Furlan D. Management of acute scrotum in children: a 25-year single center experience on 558 pediatric patients. Can J Urol. 2016;23(6):8594–601.

Ta A, D'Arcy FT, Hoag N, D'Arcy JP, Lawrentschuk N. Testicular torsion and the acute scrotum: current emergency management. Eur J Emerg Med. 2016;23(3):160–5.

119 Diagnostic Pathway: A Painful Scrotum

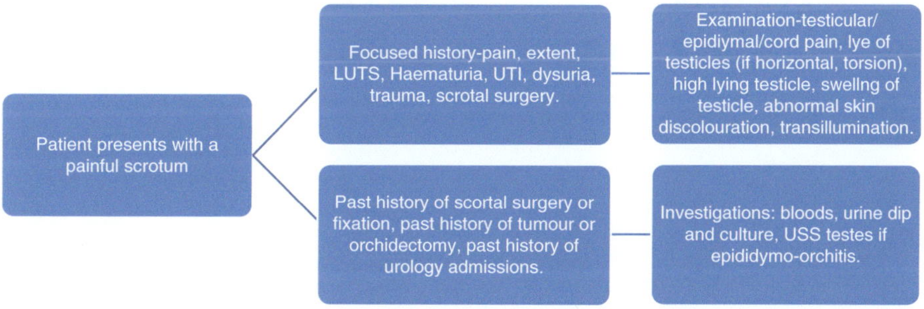

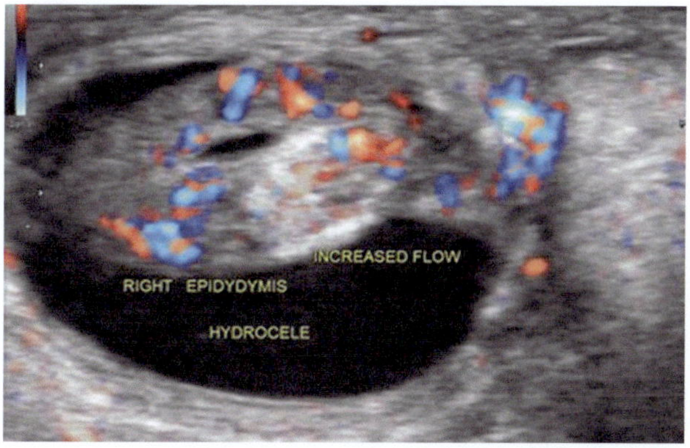

Fig. 119.1 USS of epididymo-orchitis and a hydrocele

S. S. Goonewardene et al., *Basic Urological Management*,
https://doi.org/10.1007/978-3-319-98720-0_119

Suggested Reading

D'Andrea A, Coppolino F, Cesarano E, Russo A, Cappabianca S, Genovese EA, Fonio P, Macarini L. US in the assessment of acute scrotum. Crit Ultrasound J. 2013;5(Suppl 1):S8.

Pogorelić Z, Mustapić K, Jukić M, Todorić J, Mrklić I, Mešštrović J, Jurić I, Furlan D. Management of acute scrotum in children: a 25-year single center experience on 558 pediatric patients. Can J Urol. 2016;23(6):8594–601.

Ta A, D'Arcy FT, Hoag N, D'Arcy JP, Lawrentschuk N. Testicular torsion and the acute scrotum: current emergency management. Eur J Emerg Med. 2016;23(3):160–5.

120 Management Pathway: A Painful Scrotum

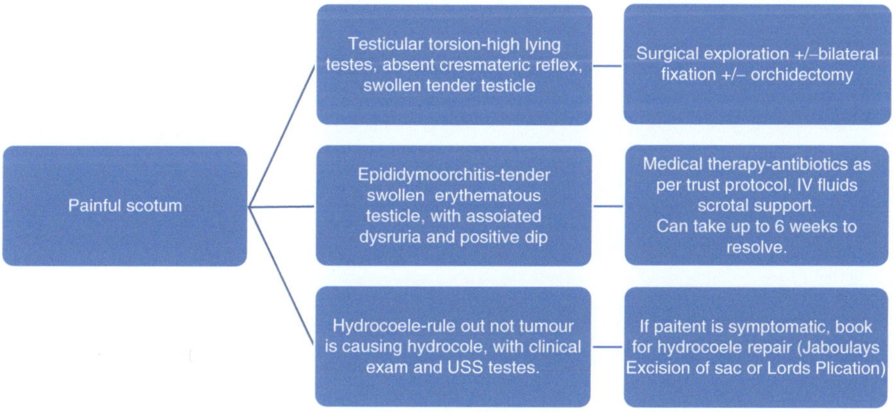

Suggested Reading

D'Andrea A, Coppolino F, Cesarano E, Russo A, Cappabianca S, Genovese EA, Fonio P, Macarini L. US in the assessment of acute scrotum. Crit Ultrasound J. 2013;5(Suppl 1):S8.

Pogorelić Z, Mustapić K, Jukić M, Todorić J, Mrklić I, Meštrović J, Jurić I, Furlan D. Management of acute scrotum in children: a 25-year single center experience on 558 pediatric patients. Can J Urol. 2016;23(6):8594–601.

Ta A, D'Arcy FT, Hoag N, D'Arcy JP, Lawrentschuk N. Testicular torsion and the acute scrotum: current emergency management. Eur J Emerg Med. 2016;23(3):160–5.

S. S. Goonewardene et al., *Basic Urological Management*,
https://doi.org/10.1007/978-3-319-98720-0_120

121 Scrotal Lesions

Definition

- A mass within the scrotum.
- This may be painful or painless with associated symptoms.
- Patients may have this for a prolonged period of time prior to realising it is present.
- It is important to rule out testicular tumour in young males, and also for tender testicles, the management of torsion.

Causes

- Benign:
- Epididymal cysts
- Hydrocele
- Varicocoele
- Testicualr cysts
- Lipoma of the cord
- inguinal hernia
- Malign
- Testicular cancer

S. S. Goonewardene et al., *Basic Urological Management*,
https://doi.org/10.1007/978-3-319-98720-0_121

History

- Extent and duration of symptoms
- Painful or Pain less
- Extent and duration of mass
- Change in mass Weight loss
- Urinary symptoms-LUTS, dysuria, haematuria, UTI, AUR
- Red flag signs-weight loss, lymphadenopaty, chest symptoms
- Prior surgery or urological history

Examination

- Obs-blood pressure, heart rate, respiratory rate
- Chest assessment-metastases or pleural effusion
- CVS assessment-? Septic
- Examination of abdomen-palpable bladder or renal mass
- Scrotal examination-pain, lesion, size, anatomical location-? abnormal testicles, transillumination (hydrocoele), cough reflex-varicocoele.

Investigation

- Bloods: FBC, renal function, crp, calcium, esr.
- USS to assess scrotal contents.
- Urine dip and culture.
- Bladder scan to assess post void residual.

Management

- Epididymal cysts-if patient has not completed family, pain relief (risk of strictures, and infertility), if family completed and patient has enlarged cyst which is symptomatic, excise.
- Hydrocele-if enlarged and patient has significant pain, list for repair, but warn against risk of recurrence.
- Varicocoele-embolise if patient is symptomatic.
- Lipoma of the cord-excise for cosmetic purposes.
- inguinal hernia-refer to general surgeons for repair.

Suggested Reading

Crawford P, Crop JA. Evaluation of scrotal masses. Am Fam Physician. 2014;89(9):723–7.
Montgomery JS, Bloom DA. The diagnosis and management of scrotal masses. Med Clin North Am. 2011;95(1):235–44.
O'Reilly P, Le J, Sinyavskaya A, Mandel ED. Evaluating scrotal masses. JAAPA. 2016;29(2):26–32.
Sommers D, Winter T. Ultrasonography evaluation of scrotal masses. Radiol Clin N Am. 2014;52(6):1265–81.

Diagnostic and Management Pathways: Scrotal Lesions

122

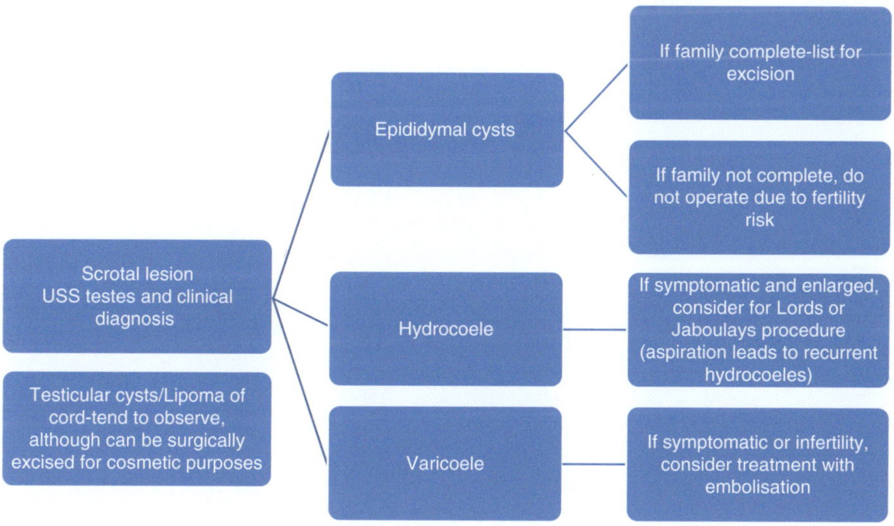

Suggested Reading

Crawford P, Crop JA. Evaluation of scrotal masses. Am Fam Physician. 2014;89(9):723–7.

Montgomery JS, Bloom DA. The diagnosis and management of scrotal masses. Med Clin North Am. 2011;95(1):235–44.

O'Reilly P, Le J, Sinyavskaya A, Mandel ED. Evaluating scrotal masses. JAAPA. 2016;29(2):26–32.

Sommers D, Winter T. Ultrasonography evaluation of scrotal masses. Radiol Clin N Am. 2014;52(6):1265–81.

S. S. Goonewardene et al., *Basic Urological Management*,
https://doi.org/10.1007/978-3-319-98720-0_122

Index

S. S. Goonewardene et al., *Basic Urological Management*,
https://doi.org/10.1007/978-3-319-98720-0

MIX
Papier aus verantwortungsvollen Quellen
Paper from responsible sources
FSC® C105338

If you have any concerns about our products,
you can contact us on
ProductSafety@springernature.com

In case Publisher is established outside the EU,
the EU authorized representative is:
Springer Nature Customer Service Center GmbH
Europaplatz 3, 69115 Heidelberg, Germany

Printed by Libri Plureos GmbH
in Hamburg, Germany